60 tips

sleep

Marie Borrel

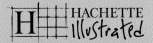

HACHETTE
Illustrated

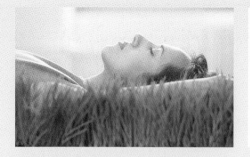
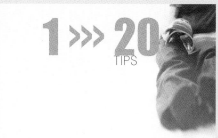

TIPS

contents

Note: The information and recommendations given in this book are not intended to be a substitute for medical advice. Consult your doctor before acting on any recommendations given in this book. The authors and publisher disclaim any liability, loss, injury or damage incurred as a consequence, directly or indirectly, of the use and application of the contents of this book.

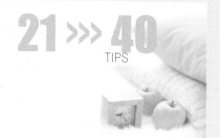

21 >>> 40
TIPS

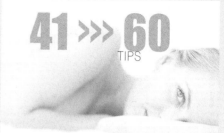

41 >>> 60
TIPS

introduction
to sleep,
perchance
to dream

The German philosopher, Friedrich Nietzsche, believed that to enjoy a good night's sleep was no small achievement and demanded that one stayed awake all day to work at it. Perhaps that is why Nietzsche is not up there with the great insomniacs, such as Napoleon and Churchill. It is true that you have to prepare for a good night's sleep in the morning and work towards it all day. All too often we forget that our sleeping hours are characterized by our daytime ones. They are imbued with the anxieties and worries of the day and affected by the food we eat and the exercise we take. Around a fifth of people say they don't sleep well, one in three actually lack sleep and a surprisingly large percentage of people take medication to help with insomnia.

Just what is insomnia?

Insomnia can cause huge problems for those unfortunate enough to suffer from it. Let's examine exactly what insomnia is. There are several issues involved but all types of insomnia have one common denominator – sufferers wake up tired and feeling they have not totally recuperated overnight. Insomnia selects its victims indiscriminately, from small children yawning on their way to school to grand-parents up and about since the crack of dawn via countless adults travelling to work with puffy eyes. Sleep specialists all agree on one point: it is important to separate insomnia proper from the conditions it triggers. It is often the feeling of disruption of our sleep patterns that is the cause of the latter.

Myth and reality

It is high time to put an end to certain long-held, preconceived ideas about insomnia. Firstly, we need to assess what constitutes 'a good night's' or 'eight-hour' sleep. We all have our own individual body clocks and different needs. Some people need only four hours a day, others cannot function with less than ten. If you belong to the first group, then you are lucky. If you need more than double the amount required by your fellow sleepers, you are not so lucky. Most people need to sleep between six and eight hours a night. Needs differ due to biological factors and these are probably hereditary, just as is our tendency either to be an early riser or a night owl. For example, we know that we tend to feel sleepy when our body temperature begins to fall but this occurs at different times according to the individual. However, individuals will experience this drop in temperature at the same time each evening and we need to respect this rhythm to maintain regular sleeping patterns.

Phases of sleep

Sleep is made up of successive phases that follow a set pattern. When we fall asleep, our brain waves gradually slow down. This state lasts between two and thirty minutes, according to the individual. We then fall into a phase of light sleep during which our body relaxes. A slow sleep phase follows which gives way after around 20 minutes to deep sleep and then very deep or profound sleep. Then comes the paradoxical phase, during which brain activity is just as important as it is during waking hours despite the fact that the body is totally inert except for REM (rapid eye movement). It is during this phase that we dream.

The cycle lasts between one and a half to two hours. We then wake up for a few seconds, falling straight back to sleep before a new cycle begins, without having the least awareness of this process.

The role of the brain

Sleep is not a voluntary act and we are at the mercy of our brain which has to slow down its electrical activity in order to take us from one phase to the next until the following morning. It is during the slow, deep sleep that we rest physically. During the paradoxical or REM phase of sleep we recuperate mentally. The phases only need to be shortened in length or intensity for the sleep to be less regenerative. We cannot issue our brains with orders but we can look after the brain by nourishing it, removing negative or draining thought, relieving unnecessary tension and administering natural remedies that don't disturb its activity. You can take these methods on board and make them part of your daily life in order to avoid disturbed sleep or help cure it. It is never too late for action.

how to use this book

●●●● FOR YOUR GUIDANCE

> A symbol at the bottom of each page will help you to identify the natural solutions available:

Herbal medicine, aromatherapy, homeopathy, Dr Bach's flower remedies – how natural medicine can help.

Simple exercises – preventing problems by strengthening your body.

Massage and manipulation – how they help to promote well-being.

Healthy eating – all you need to know about the contribution it makes.

Practical tips for your daily life – so that you can prevent instead of having to cure.

Psychology, relaxation, Zen – advice to help you be at peace with yourself and regain serenity.

> A complete programme that will solve all your health problems.
Try it!

This book offers a made-to-measure programme, which will enable you to deal with your own particular problem. It is organized into four sections:

• **A questionnaire** to help you to assess the extent of your problem.
• **The first 20 tips** that will show you how to change your daily life in order to prevent problems and maintain health and fitness.
• **20 slightly more radical tips** that will develop the subject and enable you to cope when problems occur.
• **The final 20 tips** which are intended for more serious cases, when preventative measures and attempted solutions have not worked.

At the end of each section someone with the same problem as you shares his or her experiences.

You can go methodically through the book from tip 1 to 60 putting each piece of advice into practice. Alternatively, you can pick out the recommendations which appear to be best suited to your particular case, or those which fit most easily into your daily routine. Or, finally, you can choose to follow the instructions according to whether you wish to prevent stress problems occuring or cure ones that already exist.

what sort of insomniac are you?

Read the following statements, look at the problem described, then select **A** if it rarely applies to you, **B** if it is a frequent experience and **C** if it is always the case.

A	B	C	
A	B	C	I wake up during the night and can't get back to sleep
A	B	C	I sleep badly after I have drunk alcohol with my meal
A	B	C	I worry at night about my problems
A	B	C	I have a very stressful job

A	B	C	
A	B	C	I have difficulty sleeping at night
A	B	C	I take sleeping tablets
A	B	C	I go to bed at different times
A	B	C	I have a turbulent emotional life

If you scored mostly **A**s, read Tips **1** to **20** – they offer the most suitable advice for your problems.

If you scored mostly **B**s, then go straight to Tips **21** to **40**.

If you ticked mostly **C**s, then go to Tips **41** to **60** now – it's time to take action!

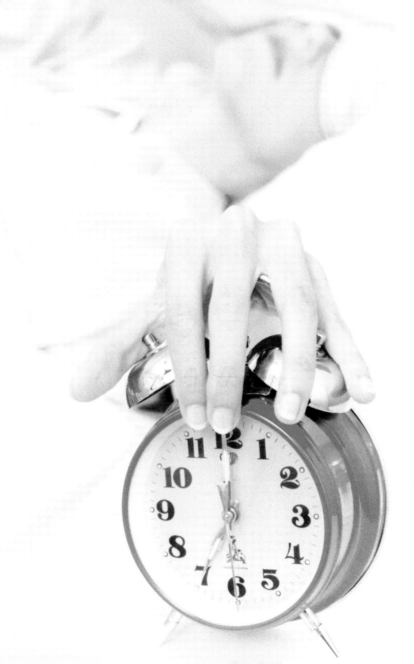

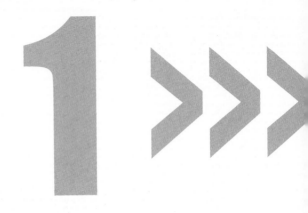

>> **Too much stress,** an unhealthy lifestyle, an unbalanced diet, lack of exercise, poor time management – all these factors can disrupt your sleeping patterns. However, a good night's sleep is the first step on the route to physical and psychological recuperation.

>>> In order to combat these problems, you should try to adopt **a good lifestyle and healthy habits**.

>>>> This section offers 20 simple, daily tips to incorporate into your life in order to **improve your sleeping pattern.**

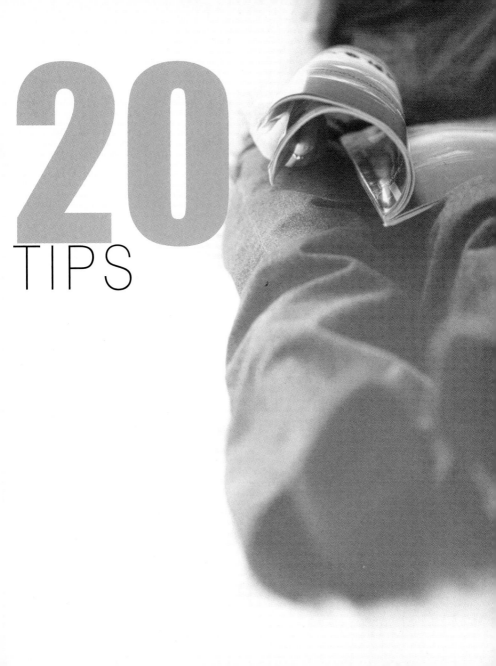

20
TIPS

If you want to encourage and maintain good sleeping habits, you must first get to know and understand them. Keeping a sleep diary or journal for a week, or even two, is an effective way of doing this. Equip yourself with a notebook and pen.

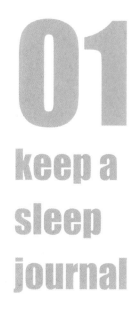

01
keep a sleep journal

Each to his or her own

We all have our own individual sleep patterns and habits, our good times and bad times. General rules and guidelines have been established through research by sleep specialists, however, each individual has his or her own peculiarities. You must understand your own before you can improve and maintain the quality of your sleep.

● ● ● DID YOU KNOW?

> You should try to sleep for eight hours each night. The most beneficial hours of sleep occur before midnight. A heavy meal can disturb your sleep.

> There are no set rules about sleep. What disrupts one person's sleep could encourage another's.

Writing it down

Equip yourself with a notebook and pen and always keep them by your bed. Make a meticulous note of every detail of your sleeping habits for at least a week or, better still, two weeks: when you feel drowsy during the day, when you want to go to bed in the evening, what you dream about, which nights you sleep well, what happened the day before, how you feel when you wake up. Gradually you will be able to draw up your own 'sleep profile'. The information will help you choose the best ways to improve your sleep and the best times to take action.

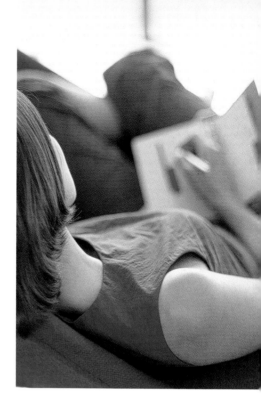

> The most important thing is to wake up full of energy whether you went to bed early or late, slept for several hours or just a few, on a full or empty stomach.

KEY FACTS

* We all have our own ways of sleeping well.

* Keep a note of all aspects of your sleeping patterns: hours, disturbances, tiredness on waking.

* Beware of paying too much attention to received ideas.

02

learn the art of bathing

There is nothing like a lovely warm bath to get you ready to slip gently into the land of nod. The heat and the contact with the water relax you naturally, both physically and mentally. It is important to understand the art of bathing.

A delicious ritual

We all spent the first nine months of our existence in a bath of warm liquid, cradled by the movements of our mother. When we slide into warm water we instantly recall the same state of happiness that provokes feelings of relaxation and sleepiness. In order to prepare yourself for a calm night's sleep, enjoy a relaxing bath but wait for at least an hour after you have eaten, in order to aid digestion.

The perfect bath

The bathroom is a room in which you can spend time alone. Lock the door, leaving behind the noise of the house and its problems. Fill the bathtub with warm water – 34 to 38°C (93 to 100°F) is the ideal temperature for relaxing your muscles whilst increasing blood and lymphatic circulation, thereby eliminating the toxins that have accumulated in the tissues through the stresses of the day. Your brain waves can synchronize at a slower pace. Spend 20 minutes in the bath, but no longer, or you will get cold or emerge with wrinkled skin like a newborn baby. Wrap yourself up in a dressing gown and head straight for bed!

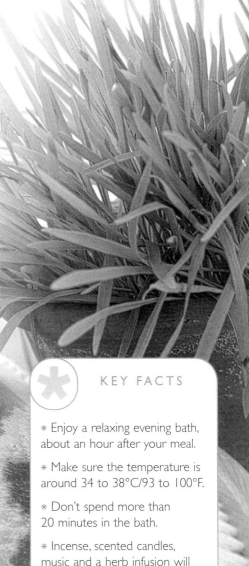

> Pour the infusion into the bath water and save a cupful to drink while you relax. Delicious!

KEY FACTS

* Enjoy a relaxing evening bath, about an hour after your meal.

* Make sure the temperature is around 34 to 38°C/93 to 100°F.

* Don't spend more than 20 minutes in the bath.

* Incense, scented candles, music and a herb infusion will help you relax.

03 focus on cereals

In order to get to sleep, your brain needs two things: a neuro-hormone serotonin and an amino acid tryptophan. Both of these are produced via carbohydrates and proteins found in food, and cereals supply all the fuel necessary to induce sleep. Tryptophan is an amino acid, one of the constituents of proteins.

●●● DID YOU KNOW?

> Vary your menus by experimenting with other cereals. Quinoa, for example, is an ancient South American whole grain and as versatile as it is nourishing.

> Add spice to your menus by cooking quinoa instead of rice, serving it with meat, fish, vegetables and spices. Why not try variations on the theme of wheat and serve bulgar wheat salad or risotto.

Brain food

The delicate transition from the state of wakefulness to that of sleep takes place in our brain. Think of it as an engine, needing fuel in order to function properly. Carbohydrates supply this vital fuel. The food we eat supplies the necessary nutrients in two forms: sugars (from sugar, honey and fruit) and cereals (pasta, rice and bread). The former are absorbed rapidly by the body which burns them on the spot. The latter are metabolized more slowly and supply our brain with fuel for longer.

Good and bad sugars

The brain consumes a large number of carbohydrates responsible for supplying it with energy, along with the rest of the body. The brain also manufactures a neuro-hormone vital to the function of sleep. This is known as serotonin and it has a calming, relaxing effect on us. A lack of serotonin in the brain will make it hard for us to switch the 'thinking engine' off. Another vital element provided by protein containing carbohydrates, such as cereals, is tryptophan, an amino acid that acts as a natural tranquillizer.

It is better to focus on cereals and limit the number of sugars you consume, in particular refined sugars such as white sugar, pastries, biscuits and sweets. Ideally, you should eat cereals in the evening in order to supply your brain with a supply on which to draw during the night. You can replenish the stock at breakfast the following morning.

KEY FACTS

* Our brain needs energy in order to function properly.

* It requires serotonin to help us make the transition between waking and sleeping.

* The brain draws vital carbohydrates from the food you eat.

* Try eating cereals at night.

> Don't forget traditional cereals such as buck-wheat. Try eating whole and organic grains in order to benefit from the vitamin content and avoid possible pesticides. Buckwheat pancakes and pasta are also delicious. Cracked wheat is delicious in pilaffs.

04

move your bed around

The quality of your sleep can also depend on the position and location of your bed, according to geobiologists. They maintain that the earth is traversed by electromagnetic lines and that we should avoid their intersection points if we want to enjoy a good night's sleep.

Dr Hartmann's discovery

The term 'geobiology' was first used by Dr Hartmann, a German doctor and researcher (1915-1992). He documented the existence of electromagnetic rays emanating from the earth. Hartmann maintained that the earth is traversed by a kind of network or grid of invisible lines that run north to south or east to west, around 2 metres (just over 6 feet) apart, in a net-like formation. Where the lines intersect, the rays

ZZZZ

– in themselves not harmful – are amplified. If you sleep for too long over one of these so-called 'telluric' or 'Hartmann knots', your sleep may become disturbed.

Detective work

There are two solutions to this problem. The simplest of these is to move your bed around at least every two years. It takes several years for the 'Hartmann knots' to disrupt sleep patterns. The second option involves detective work on your part. Equip yourself with a portable radio, tune it to shortwave between two stations and you will be able to detect the crackling noises. Proceed to the next room on a north-south axis. If the noise decreases you are on a Hartmann line. Put a marker on the floor and do the same for an east-west axis. Simply note the point at which the lines intersect – this is the location of the knots to be avoided. What you are looking for is a geobiologically neutral place.

● ● ● DID YOU KNOW?

> A geobiologist is a 'house doctor', interested not only in the Hartmann grid but also in the subterranean layout. An expert in the field will trace the underground water channels and track sources of electrical pollution hidden around the house. Like any other therapist, he or she will diagnose the problem and suggest treatment, which in this case may include moving furniture and insulating (or isolating) certain electrical installations. The goal is to ensure that the house does not have a negative impact on those living in it.

KEY FACTS

* The earth is surrounded by a network of electro-magnetic rays, something like a ball in a net.

* Avoid sleeping for too long in a spot where the lines intersect.

* Change your bed around at least every two years.

* Ask a geobiologist to advise you on the ideal position for your bed.

05

air your room

You will have a much better night's sleep if you breathe in pure air. Make sure you sleep in a properly aired room, void of fustiness, fumes and other forms of pollution. Transform your nights with one simple action – open the window for one hour a day.

Vital nourishment

Of all the things that nourish us as humans, oxygen is the most vital. We can last a few weeks without eating, several days without drinking but only a few minutes without breathing. Each one of our millions of cells needs a constant supply of oxygen in order to function properly and execute the countless biochemical operations vital for our

●●● DID YOU KNOW?

> Despite what many may think, sleeping with the window open is not generally to be recommended, particularly for those living in large towns or cities.

Changes in temperature can disturb sleep, and noise can be disruptive even if it does not actually wake you up. The smells and lights of the streets do not do much to help.

survival. The air we breathe supplies us with this precious element. Breathing regulates our nervous system and relaxes our minds – two key factors involved in the quality and quantity of sleep we enjoy. This air should be of the best quality possible.

Breathe clean air

Rooms that are not properly aired can become stale. The level of oxygen diminishes whilst that of carbon gases increases. The temperature also plays an important role. If the room is too warm, we wake up and experience difficulty in getting back to sleep. If it is too cold, the most regenerative phase of sleep, the REM (Rapid Eye Movement) phase, can be disrupted. The ideal temperature for healthy and natural sleep is around 17 to 18°C (63 to 65°F). Make sure that you air your bedrooms properly. Open the windows as wide as possible in the morning and leave them open for at least ten minutes, the amount of time required to renew the air in an average-sized bedroom. Repeat this operation in the evening, around half an hour before you retire.

KEY FACTS

* Breathing clean, healthy air is vital for the relaxation of our nervous system.

* Air your bedroom regularly, both morning and night.

* The ideal temperature of your bedroom is between 17 to 18°C (63 to 65°F).

* Don't sleep with your bedroom window open.

06

fill your lungs with oxygen

We are good at breathing badly and need to relearn how to breathe deeply and effectively using our abdomen, just as we did when we were babies. Proper breathing enables our cells to recuperate and our bodies to relax and sleep.

The bridge between the brain and the body

You may be surprised to discover that we breathe no fewer than 20,000 times a day. It is the only vital bodily function that is both conscious and unconscious. During the night, when we are asleep, we continue to breathe without thinking about it. However, if we want to control our breathing, we can do so at any time. We can speed it up, slow it down or hold it at will. In this way our breathing represents a bridge between the brain and

● ● ● DID YOU KNOW? ────────────

> The nose plays a vital role in the breathing process. It warms and moistens the oxygen as it travels through its passages, stripping it of dust and grime at the same time.

> The nose is also equipped with a mucus lining that humidifies the air as it is inhaled.

the body, the mental and the physical. Learning to breathe deeply helps us to control our emotions, reduce feelings of anxiety and prepare for a calm sleep.

Breathing through your stomach

Abdominal breathing helps to improve the exchange of gases by forcing air deep into the alveoli (air cells). Waste matter is dispelled more quickly and effectively and our body is cleansed. This relaxed form of breathing helps dispel nerves and relieve tension and stress. Follow the instructions below and perform this breathing exercise for a few minutes just before going to bed. It will help you prepare for sleep.
• Breathe in whilst inflating your stomach and then your thoracic cage.
• Count to five whilst retaining the oxygen in your lungs.
• Exhale slowly whilst contracting your abdominal muscles.
• Count to five before inhaling again.

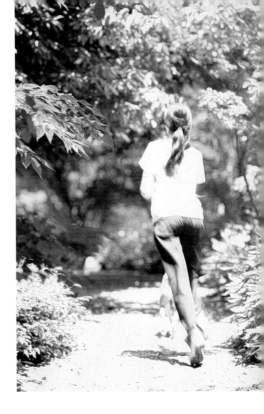

> It is also armed with cilia (nasal hairs) that capture the particles of dust and then expel them during exhalation.

KEY FACTS

* Breathing properly helps relieve tension and reduce stress.

* Take large, deep breaths using your abdominal muscles.

* Breathe deeply before going to sleep.

07

choose your bed carefully

Soft or hard mattress? Natural or synthetic fibres? Slats or springs? The quality of your bed plays an important role in the quality of your sleep, even your life. Remember that you spend one third of your lifetime in your bed. It's important to choose the right one.

Twenty years in bed

Question: how do we spend around a third of our lifetime, which on average equals between 20 and 25 years? Answer: asleep. And that's not all – your waking hours can also suffer as a result of poor sleep. A lack of sleep can affect all aspects of your life and at the heart of this issue lies, quite literally, the quality of your bed. A good bed is one in which you feel good. It is important to avoid mattresses that are too soft as they will not support your spine properly. Excessively hard mattresses are often uncomfortable. If you suffer from a bad back, go for the harder rather than the softer option.

Bedtime rules

• **The mattress:** Avoid woollen mattresses as they are high-maintenance and need to be turned once a week. If you prefer foam mattresses, choose a good quality one, in natural latex if possible and at least 20-cm (8-inches) thick. If you opt for a mattress with springs, check exactly how many there are. More springs equals more effective support. There can be anywhere between 200 and 2,000 in different brands.

• **The base:** a base with interconnecting slats is both the most comfortable and efficient option. It adapts to the shape of your body and your movements during sleep.

• **The pillow:** avoid sleeping with your head too elevated. It can damage your cervical vertebrae. Ergonomic pillows that are specially designed to protect your spine are now widely available.

> They do not like synthetic fibres as much as natural ones, so take the synthetic option if you suffer from allergies. Washing, vital for removing the parasites, is much easier.

KEY FACTS

∗ The quality of sleep depends on the quality of the bed.

∗ Your bed should be neither too hard nor too soft.

∗ If you suffer from a bad back, go for a firm mattress rather than a soft one.

∗ Choose natural fibres over synthetic ones, unless you suffer from allergies.

08 respect the routine

You will not sleep well if others fail to respect your routine. You need others to participate in your sleep programme if it is to succeed.

The temple of sleep A bedroom is not a living area, television room or office. It is certainly not a games room. The bedroom should be a temple of sleep. Take a leaf out of your pet's book – find a spot (a nest or burrow would be the wild animal equivalent) used exclusively for sleep and a no-go area for others. Animals have the right idea, naturally.

Sleep programme If your bedroom is used exclusively for the purpose of sleep, just entering it in the evening will trigger a sort of automatic reflex that prepares your body and mind for sleep. Some action on your part will help reinforce the concept of your bedroom as a sleep sanctuary, as follows:

• Try not to set up your home office in the bedroom. If you have no choice, separate the area with a screen or book case.
• Make your bedroom a no-smoking area.
• Try to ensure the house is quiet when you are sleeping.
• Teach your children or housemates to respect the sleep routine of others if they are the first to wake up in the house.

●●● DID YOU KNOW?

> If you have noisy neighbours, go and speak to them about your sleep problems. Don't be aggressive or critical, simply inform them of your sleep routine – what time you go to bed and when you wake up during the night. You can then come to a mutually acceptable arrangement.

KEY FACTS

✳ Your bedroom is not an office, living room, games room or smoking area.

✳ Teach those you live with to respect your sleep routine.

09 avoid disturbing visual images

Your bedroom is not a cinema! Watch the TV in the living room and try not to have a set in the bedroom at all. Choose your evening viewing options carefully.

Stress and sleep don't make good bedfellows If you are anxious, stressed or nervous, sleep will come less easily and may not be deep or restorative. Negative, dark thoughts can cause violent dreams that disrupt sleep. It's difficult to dismiss the stresses and strains of life from your thoughts. Work problems, financial worries, relationship and family difficulties don't just disappear at night. However, avoid making things worse by watching disturbing images late in the evening and try to think things over or make decisions early in the evening.

Happy endings, happy nights Firstly, ban the television set from the bedroom. If you really want to watch something potentially disturbing, do so in the living room. Sleeping in a different room will create a distance between the images you have seen and your night's sleep. This separation of locations is important. Try to create a positive atmosphere in the evenings before heading off to bed.

● ● ● DID YOU KNOW?

> If violent images linger in your head as you are about to retire, try a few simple relaxation techniques before actually going to bed. Lie down, close your eyes, breathe deeply and slowly, and imagine that you are gradually dispelling all the disturbing images through your nostrils as you exhale.

KEY FACTS

* Ban the television set from your bedroom.

* Avoid watching violent or depressing films.

* Try a method of relaxation before retiring if you feel disturbed by distressing visual images.

10

redecorate your room

Feng shui is an ancient Chinese discipline based on the concept of the harmonization of energy as a form of 'medicine' or treatment. Its fundamental principles can be applied to the bedroom in order to improve sleeping patterns and avoid disruption.

Harmonization of energy

Feng shui can be applied to all areas and aspects of the home, including location and position together with interior décor and the placement of doors and windows. For the Chinese, the house in which one lives exercises an importance influence over our health and inner balance and, as a result, our sleep. Chinese traditional thinking maintains

●●● DID YOU KNOW?

> Feng shui helps to establish a balance between yin and yang, the two complementary elements that make up vital energy.

> Yin is feminine, dark, liquid, passive and cold whilst its counterpart, yang, is masculine, bright, solid, active and warm.

that energy is all around us, omnipresent. It is within all living organisms and circulates in our habitat. Feng shui regulates and harmonizes energy within the home just as acupuncture works on the body.

The ideal bedroom

• **Sharp angles:** avoid furniture with pointed, angular features, as these introduce negative energy. This is particularly the case if any points are directed towards the bed.
• **Houseplants:** if you like plants, choose round-leafed varieties and place them in a westerly or north-westerly position where they can be most effective in promoting sleep.
• **Curtains:** invest in double-thickness curtains. The heavy fabric slows down the circulation of energy and calms you

as you sleep as well as cutting out light and noise.
• **Mirrors:** remove any mirrors from you bedroom, particularly if you have one facing the bed. They reflect the sleeper's vital energy and bounce back negative emotions that may be dispelled during sleep.
• **Smooth surfaces and hard materials:** avoid marble and glass in the bedroom as they accelerate the circulation of energy and can disrupt sleep.

> Efficient and positive circulation of energy relies on the perfect balance of yin and yang.

KEY FACTS

* Feng shui harmonizes the circulation of energy within the home.

* You need to slow down the energy in order to sleep well.

* Avoid mirrors, sharp angles, pointed objects, smooth surfaces and hard materials.

* Make sure you invest in some thick, heavy curtains.

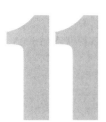

11
find time for sport and exercise

Exercise helps you sleep. Try and choose an enjoyable, convenient form of physical exercise or a sport that suits your ability. Don't overdo it. Too much exercise can be as detrimental as none at all.

Sport is good for everyone – well, almost

Regular physical exercise is the best thing you can do to maintain your figure, your health and the quality of your sleep. It improves the oxygenation of cells, increases your respiratory capacity and helps expels toxins. It relieves nervous tensions, reduces anxiety and can go some way to dispelling negative thoughts. Exercise also tires out the

● ● ● DID YOU KNOW?

> Try your hand at rollerblading. It is very trendy, it's an endurance sport and combines efficient transport with effective exercise. Long stretches at a relatively moderate speed are as beneficial as walking, jogging or cycling.

> Do note, however, that in big towns and cities you will breathe in all the traffic fumes and pollution, which will fill your lungs. Wear a mask or try rollerblading in parks and gardens instead.

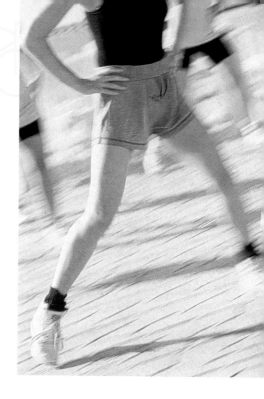

body thereby relaxing your mind. However, make sure you don't overdo it – if you are too tired physically then you may find it difficult to get to sleep and have a disrupted night.

Where, when and how?

It is important for you to enjoy your exercise for it to help you sleep properly. If it is just another entry on your list of things to do, an additional source of stress, it will not encourage a good night's slumber.

• Try to choose an outdoor sport in order to get as much oxygen into your system as possible.

• Whatever form of exercise you select, make sure you practise it regularly without forcing or exhausting yourself. Twice a week for forty minutes is about the minimum amount you should do.

• Choose a sport that works the whole body, such as walking, swimming, jogging (but not too fast) or cycling.

• Don't exercise just before going to bed. Wait for at least half an hour before you retire.

• Don't forget to drink plenty of water in order to help dispel the toxins from your system. A 'clean' body sleeps more easily.

 KEY FACTS

* Sport helps you sleep better.

* Exercise regularly without forcing yourself.

* Don't play sport or exercise just before going to bed.

* Try rollerblading in green spaces, well away from pollution and traffic fumes.

12 drink plenty of water

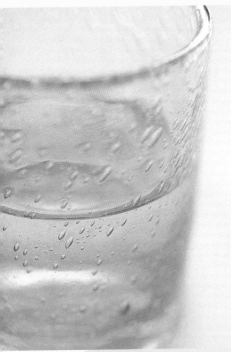

There's no life without water. We need to drink to keep the body hydrated, to nourish our cells and to evacuate toxins. But we also need water if we are to sleep soundly, because a dehydrated body finds it difficult to sleep.

DID YOU KNOW?

> Water softeners and purifiers do not actually affect the mineral content of tap water but they do get rid of some undesirable substances, such as nitrates (these are minerals and hard water is a useful source of calcium). Nitrates can damage your health if taken in

No water, no rest!

Our body is 70% water. It has to be constantly replenished because it is this water that ensures that nutrients are carried to the cells (via the arteries) and that toxins are transported to the excreting organs (via the lymph system and veins). We need to drink at least 1½ litres (2½ pints) of water a day.

Sleep quickly suffers if we do not drink enough liquid. A badly drained body suffers insidious fatigue, which disrupts rest. The electrical activity of a dehydrated brain quickly loses its intensity and some brain functions can 'come to a standstill', particularly the ability to move from a state of wakefulness to one of sleep.

Choose your water carefully

Tap water is usually drinkable – it is healthy in bacteriological terms. However, its composition varies greatly from one region to another, being more or less rich in mineral salts depending on the terrain it has passed through. This is particularly true in the case of magnesium and calcium, which are essential for the nervous system. If you prefer mineral waters, it is important to note that spring waters do not have any recognized therapeutic qualities and that they can vary in composition depending on the time of year. Some mineral waters, on the other hand, are awarded certificates recognizing their therapeutic qualities depending on their mineral salt content. Their composition must be constant and is shown in detail on the label.

large quantities that exceed the limits that the body can tolerate. This can be the case in some agricultural regions.

KEY FACTS

* Drink 1½ litres (2½ pints) of water per day to evacuate toxins and nourish your cells.

* A dehydrated body chokes up with waste and becomes tired, which leads to disturbed sleep and brain activity.

* Some mineral waters are particularly rich in magnesium and calcium.

13

try an infusion

Our grandmothers had a penchant for an evening infusion, such as verbena, lime or camomile. These digestive, soothing and calming infusions gently prepared them for sleep. Why not follow their example?

The secrets of a successful infusion

An evening infusion is more of a ritual than a therapeutic act. After the evening meal, prepare a drink to enjoy with family or friends. Many of the plants now used for this convivial custom have left the confines of the medicine cabinet for the supermarket shelves, but they are no less effective.

It is best not to add sugar to infusions. That way, you avoid having too much

● ● ● DID YOU KNOW?

> Infusions are usually made from dried plants, which are more effective. The active constituents are contained in vegetal cells, the walls of which are made of cellulose.

> When the plant is fresh, even boiling water cannot break down the cellulose, so some of the active constituents remain in the plant.

sugar in your diet, and glucose digestion does not then interfere with the assimilation of the infusion's active constituents. You can add a little honey instead.

Evening infusions

• **Lime** is a tranquilizer that improves sleep and eases digestion troubles associated with stress. You can drink it throughout the day, because its calming properties are very mild. Use 1 teaspoonful per cup; leave to infuse for 10 minutes.

• **Lemon balm** can be helpful in times of stress. It has a calming effect, aids digestion and tones the body to help it resist tension. Use 1 tablespoonful per 250 ml (8 fl oz) of water; leave to infuse for 10 minutes.

• **Camomile** calms, sooths and relieves tension and its accompanying aches and pains. Use 1 tablespoonful per 250 ml (8 fl oz) of water; leave to infuse for 10 minutes.

• **Verbena** calms the mind, preparing it for sleep. Use 1 teaspoonful per cup of water; leave to infuse for 10 minutes.

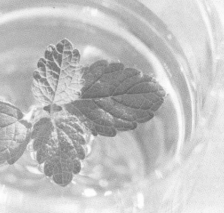

> But if the plant is dried, the drying process breaks down the cellulose, so that all the beneficial substances can pass through the cell walls into the water.

14 enjoy a warm footbath

There's nothing worse than cold feet. Sometimes they are enough on their own to disturb sleep. One simple solution is to warm up the extremities with a warm footbath.

Thyroid trouble: it is very difficult to drift off to sleep when we feel 'chilled to the marrow' and our extremities are frozen. This phenomenon is sometimes due to a lazy thyroid gland. Your doctor can easily confirm the diagnosis with a blood test and treatment with thyroid hormone is very straightforward. Most cold feet are not due to any specific cause and the thing to do in this case is to regulate these minor daily irritations by means of natural methods.

Cooking salt, seaweed or essential oils: A warm footbath is the simplest solution. All you have to do is fill a bowl with water heated to 39°C (102°F), so just a few degrees above the average internal body temperature. You can then add a handful of seaweed or a few drops of essential oil to scent or soften the water. Plunge your feet into this bath for ten minutes, then wrap them in a towel, but do not rub them dry. Go to bed as soon as they are dry.

● ● ● DID YOU KNOW?

> Circulation problems, especially arterial disease, can cause cold feet. In this case, it's best to avoid warm footbaths, as poor circulation cannot carry the heat away and there's a risk of scalding the skin. The same goes for a hot water bottle. In this case try a foot massage or even bedsocks.

KEY FACTS

＊ It's sometimes difficult to get off to sleep when your feet are icy cold.

＊ A warm footbath can help in this case.

15 establish a regular bedtime routine

Our body is a creature of habit, and sleep is no exception to this rule. A precondition of any tactic to combat insomnia is to determine the bedtime that is right for you and to stick to it.

The vicious circle: it's important to respect the body's natural rhythms if we are to stay in good health. When we don't get enough sleep or sleep badly, we quickly become trapped in a vicious circle: tiredness builds up, causing disturbed nights. One of the first things to do to try to regain a balance is to go to bed at the same time each night, and no matter how badly you sleep, to get up at the same time each day, and don't try to catch up on sleep in the middle of the day or you won't feel tired at bed time.

The best time is the time that's right for you. The best time to go to bed is the time that enables you to sleep well and to wake full of energy. Your sleep journal (see pages 12–13) will help you to determine the right time. Try to stick to it for at least a month. Once the rhythm is established, you can bend the rules slightly every now and again.

● ● ● DID YOU KNOW?

> Office and school hours mean that our social life is best suited to 'larks' rather than 'night-owls'. If you have to get up early, try to establish a bedtime that is right for you and your sleep, and takes into account what you are doing – then stick to it.

KEY FACTS

* Respect your biorhythms: the best time to go to bed is the time that will enable you to sleep well and wake up full of energy.

* Stick to the same bedtime for at least a month.

16

take a siesta

We know that our biorhythms predispose us to two segments of sleep in twenty-four hours: a long one during the night and a short one after lunch. If you have an overwhelming desire to sleep in the early afternoon, then treat yourself to a little siesta.

One of life's sweetest pleasures

It's hard to beat the pleasure of a siesta in the heat of a summer's afternoon, lulled by the chirruping of the birds and the dust motes dancing in the rays of sunlight filtering through the shutters. A siesta is a luxury we usually only allow ourselves on holiday, after a rather too boozy lunch. And that is where we go wrong: a few minutes' shut-eye early in the afternoon will not disturb our sleep at night – in fact quite the opposite.

● ● ● DID YOU KNOW?

> We have two 'sleep peaks' a day: at night, around two or three o'clock in the morning, and in the afternoon, at about two or three o'clock, when we are likely to have an energy dip.

> Various studies have shown that it is beneficial to acknowledge these two natural 'peaks'.

A siesta does not need to be long to be refreshing. Half an hour will do and more is probably too much. An afternoon nap is an effective way of improving the balance between the sympathetic and parasympathetic nervous systems, whilst helping to remove stress and tension. It also prevents a build-up of tiredness, which disturbs night-time sleep.

The art of the mini-siesta

Salvador Dali used to doze in an armchair holding a small spoon in his hand. As soon as he dropped off, his muscles relaxed and the spoon fell to the ground, waking him up. Although he was asleep for only a few seconds, it was enough to refresh him. To put it more simply, you can easily learn to fall asleep for a few minutes, just sitting in a chair or on a sofa. That is often all you need to restart the day on a good footing, leaving you less tired right through to the evening.

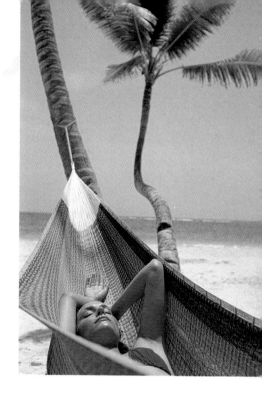

> These studies are corroborated by observations made on potholers who stayed down caves for several weeks, deprived of their usual reference points (such as time and light). Their sleep naturally fell into two periods: a long one at night and a short one during the day.

 KEY FACTS

* The desire to sleep in the middle of the day is in keeping with our biorhythms.

* A siesta will not disturb night-time sleep – in fact the opposite is true.

* Try mini-siestas: just a few minutes is often enough.

17 avoid stimulants

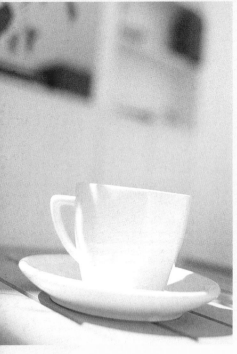

Coffee, tobacco and alcohol are guaranteed to deprive you of a good night's sleep. To prepare yourself for calm and restful nights, you really must limit your intake of such stimulants, or better still, cut them out altogether.

> Some constituents of tobacco are also stimulants, which promote fast-flowing streams of thought that are difficult to calm down.

> There are several reasons why you should cut out tobacco as well as coffee.

The most harmful stimulant: coffee

The Arab word 'kawa', sometimes used to describe the bitter, black beverage, is derived from a Brazilian term meaning 'kills sleep'. And it's true: the caffeine contained in coffee reduces the duration of our nights and disturbs deep sleep (the most recuperative). Consumed in large quantities, coffee upsets the balance of the nervous system. People who drink a lot of coffee are often locked in a vicious circle: their sleep is disturbed, so they wake feeling tired and therefore drink more coffee to keep themselves awake during the day, making the next night even more difficult.

Drink no more than two or three cups a day, none after 4 p.m., and don't make it too strong. Opt for Arabica coffee, which contains less caffeine than the Robusta beans. Remember, too, that many fizzy drinks contain caffeine, and a cup of tea contains about half the caffeine of a cup of coffee. Caffeine also has a diuretic effect. Drinking tea or coffee late in the evening can result in waking up in the night to pass water.

> Smoke inhalation damages the lungs and makes breathing less effective. Nicotine in smoke has a direct effect on neuro-transmitters in the brain and may affect sleep.

Alcohol makes you sleepy, but…

Alcohol acts differently. It is a depressant to the central nervous system and it causes a loss of inhibition. As the level rises in the blood stream, people feel tired and sleepy. However, the total period of sleep is shortened and, most importantly, is of poorer quality. Excess alcohol reduces the period of REM sleep, which is when we dream. Alcohol is burned off at the rate of one glass of wine an hour. When it has left the blood stream people feel wide awake. It also has a diuretic action. Avoid strong alcoholic drinks and content yourself with a good red wine (no more than two glasses a day for women and three for men), which has the benefit of containing antioxidants, which protects against the effects of ageing. Always try and drink a glass of water for every glass of wine.

KEY FACTS

* Drink no more than two or three cups of coffee a day (preferably Arabica).

* Avoid strong alcohol and drink no more than three glasses of good red wine a day.

* Try to cut out tobacco.

18

The more relaxed you are, the better you will sleep. It's also important to find the inner calm that helps us sleep. To relax effectively, treat yourself to a little relaxation session before you go to bed.

treat yourself to a relaxation session

Think about something else

To drift smoothly from a state of wakefulness to one of sleep, the body must be relaxed and the mind calm. If we are mulling over problems and worries or our muscles are tied up in knots due to stress, we are never going to reach the land of nod. The solution is simple: learn to relax.

There are many forms of relaxation. Some are mental, others physical.

● ● ● DID YOU KNOW?

> At the beginning of the twentieth century, Edmund Jacobson (1885-1976) developed a method of relaxation that involved contracting the muscles and then releasing them.

> Noticing these tensions helps us to relax our muscles consciously, making for deeper and more effective relaxation.

Some methods calm the emotions, others involve escaping into the world of the imagination. But they are all based on the same principle: breathing, relaxing your body and focusing your attention on 'something else'.

Guided tour

Stretched out on your bed, in the peaceful darkness, breathe deeply for several minutes, then focus your attention on your feet. When you can really 'feel' them, relax all the muscles in your feet. Then move on to your legs, your knees, thighs, pelvis, stomach and chest, and go right along your arms to your hands. Then, starting from the base of your spine, work up along the backbone to the neck and the skull; then work down over the face to the jaw. You will probably have fallen asleep before you complete this circuit.

Breathing is an essential tool of relaxation. To focus your thoughts on your body, try to become aware of your breath as it enters and leaves your nostrils. This initial exercise will help you relax. Sometimes it's enough on its own to get you to sleep.

KEY FACTS

* To sleep well, it is important that we are relaxed both physically and mentally.

* Learn to relax in bed at night before you go to sleep.

* Breathing is an essential tool of relaxation.

19

find a quiet place

It's an intrusive enemy, a permanent nuisance that eats away at our sleep even if we are unaware of it. Noise is the number one complaint as far as the environment is concerned. It is the curse of modern urban living. Learn to cut yourself off from noise nuisance.

Say no to night-time noise nuisance

The problem of noise is not always an easy one to solve. However, silence – even if it is only relative – is an essential condition of good sleep. Some people are subjected to a noisy environment all day long (traffic noise or the hum of machinery, for example) leading to nervous fatigue, so they would need even more silence than other people the following night.

Noise causes major physiological disturbances to the body, including the neuromuscular, circulatory and hormonal systems.

Night-time noise is particularly intrusive as there are fewer outside distractions.

Anti-noise solutions

The ideal solution is to soundproof your bedroom. However, this is often an onerous task and sometimes presents technical difficulties. If you live in a very noisy urban environment, the least you can do is install double glazing. Thick curtains, which absorb the noise from outside, and wallpaper, which will prevent the noise from resonating, are additional options.

If the noise comes from your neighbours (and if it is intolerable), have no compunction about contacting one of the many associations that campaign against noise – they will be happy to help you deal with the problem.

Finally, remember good old-fashioned earplugs. They may take a little getting used to, but they can provide a simple, cheap and effective solution. Listening to music played quietly may also help by distracting you.

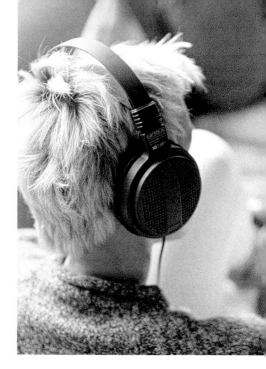

KEY FACTS

∗ Noise is the main nuisance as far as the environment is concerned. It disturbs us both physically and psychologically.

∗ Soundproof your bedroom, install double glazing and think about getting thick curtains and wallpapering your bedroom.

∗ Remember to try good old-fashioned earplugs.

20 put hops in your pillow

Old-fashioned recipes are sometimes right. It has long been known that breathing in hop-scented air promotes calm and sound sleep. Fill a pillow with hops for a guaranteed result.

It's all in the smell: hops are not just good for making beer — they also have sedative qualities. The hop cone (the cluster of flowers) contains lupulin, an essential oil that contains various active constituents, some of which have a sedative effect. The simple fact of breathing in these active constituents helps you to fall asleep.

Pillow plus infusion: stuff a small pillow with hop cones, taking care not to overfill it as otherwise it will be too firm. Change the stuffing every three or four weeks. To make this natural method more effective, drink a hop infusion at night before going to bed: use 10 g (¹/₃ oz) per 250 ml (8 fl oz) of water; leave to infuse for 10 minutes.

KEY FACTS

* Stuff a small pillow with some hop cones.

* Hop cones are full of a volatile essential oil that promotes sleep.

* Drink an infusion of hops at night before going to bed.

case study

'I'm quite a good patient: I'm fairly resistant to illness and I don't complain. But there are two things that I just cannot bear: toothache and insomnia. When I start waking up during the night, I get into an incredible nervous state. I calculate the sleep I am losing; I anticipate just how tired I will be in when I get up and just how difficult the day ahead will be. It's a real nightmare!

Fortunately, it doesn't happen that often. But, there again, I do what I can to make sure that it doesn't. I prefer to use natural methods. So I have found out how to maintain good sleep. I can tell you how it works: I drink water that is rich in magnesium; I have changed my bed; I don't drink any coffee after two o'clock in the afternoon; I have had my bedroom windows soundproofed and I have adopted a regular sleeping pattern. And above all, twice a week I treat myself to a bath fit for a queen just before I go to bed: music, candles, incense and so on.

It's wonderful — I sleep like a baby.'

21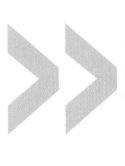

>> All it takes is a major work worry, a sudden change in your family situation or even a sudden improvement in your living conditions, and **your nights become tinged with new problems.**

>>>> Age also disrupts sleeping habits **but there's no need to exaggerate things.** It's true – lack of sleep is definitely tiring but not as much as we sometimes think. The distress caused by the decreased number of hours of sleep and the fear of being tired are often more worrying than the actual lack of sleep itself.

>>>>>> And that is a point worth thinking about before you put into practice the following 20 tips on how to **deal with occasional insomnia.**

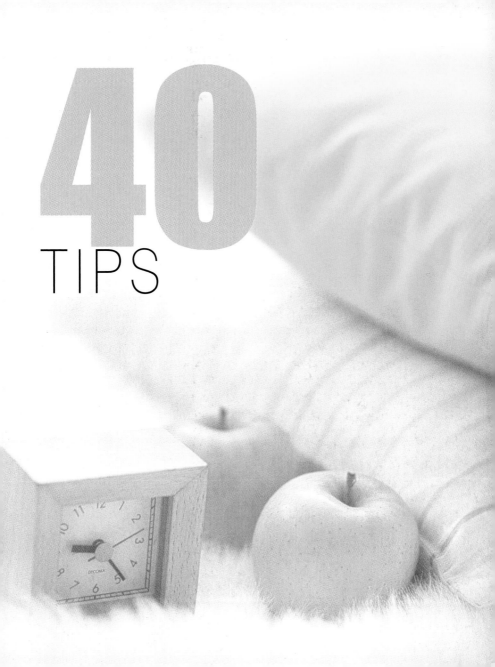

40
TIPS

21
learn the importance of vitamin B

B-group vitamins are essential if the brain and the nervous system are to function properly. If you lack these vitamins, you will become irritable, nervous, sometimes even aggressive. And sleep will be the first thing to suffer.

Vitamins for the nervous system

Each B-group vitamin has different properties: B1 protects against anxiety and improves the passage of nervous influxes between the brain cells; B2 protects against the effects of stress; B3 is involved in synthesizing the hormones that promote sleep; B5 relieves fatigue; B6 and B9 improve the emotional balance, whilst B12 helps the entire nervous system to function properly.

● ● ● DID YOU KNOW?

> B-group vitamins are water-soluble, so there is no risk of overdose: if you do take too much, you will pass out the excess in your urine.

> If you smoke or drink alcohol regularly, increase the recommended doses of B-group vitamins slightly, because these 'bad habits' mean you will need more.

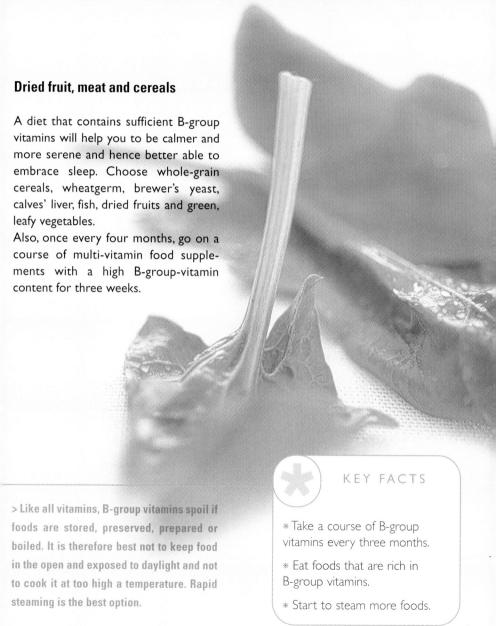

Dried fruit, meat and cereals

A diet that contains sufficient B-group vitamins will help you to be calmer and more serene and hence better able to embrace sleep. Choose whole-grain cereals, wheatgerm, brewer's yeast, calves' liver, fish, dried fruits and green, leafy vegetables.

Also, once every four months, go on a course of multi-vitamin food supplements with a high B-group-vitamin content for three weeks.

> Like all vitamins, B-group vitamins spoil if foods are stored, preserved, prepared or boiled. It is therefore best not to keep food in the open and exposed to daylight and not to cook it at too high a temperature. Rapid steaming is the best option.

KEY FACTS

* Take a course of B-group vitamins every three months.

* Eat foods that are rich in B-group vitamins.

* Start to steam more foods.

22

enjoy
essential oils

Extremely volatile, essential oils evaporate into the atmosphere, thus diffusing their calming active constituents. When we breathe them in, they penetrate into our lungs and spread throughout the body.

Sleep concentrates

Essential oils are extracts from aromatic plants. The active constituents are up to one hundred times more concentrated in the essential oil than in the living plant. Each oil has more than a dozen active constituents (rosemary has up to 250!). Each oil can have different properties, depending on the plant it was extracted from. Some have a sedative effect,

● ● ● DID YOU KNOW?

> Avoid synthetic or semi-synthetic oils. They are mere chemical copies of the real oils. They do not have the same therapeutic qualities of the natural essences and can cause unpleasant reactions, such as itching and nausea.

> Choose oils that are 100% natural (blends of several essences) or 100% pure and natural (just one essence).

calming and promoting sleep. Just diffuse them in the air to reap their benefits. The active constituents then penetrate into the respiratory system and pass into the blood through the fine walls of the pulmonary alveoli (air sacs in the lungs). The circulatory system then sees to it that the oil's active constituents reach all the cells.

Diffusers or terracotta discs

You can get yourself an essential oil diffuser: this is a small electrical appliance that slowly diffuses the essential oil throughout the room. You can also get terracotta discs. Place a disc above the light bulb of a lamp and sprinkle it with essential oils. When the lamp is lit, the heat speeds up the evaporation of the active constituents.

All essential oils are bactericides and so purify the ambient atmosphere. The following essential oils are best for promoting sleep: camomile, lemon balm, lime, rosemary, sandalwood, ylang ylang, lavender, bergamot, rosewood, jasmine, orange, citronella, neroli and mandarin.

> The very best oils are 100% pure and natural, organic and obtained from plants cultivated without the use of pesticides or chemical fertilizers.

KEY FACTS

* Essential oils diffuse their active constituents into the air.

* They have a calming effect that promotes sleep.

* They purify the air.

* It is best to choose pure and natural essential oils.

23 breathe clean air

The air we breathe contains electric particles called ions. Some are positive, others negative. It is the negative ions that are beneficial to our health and sleep.

Town ions… When we take a walk in the countryside, the air is full of beneficial negative ions. But in towns, atmospheric pollution destroys these fragile ions and increases the number of positive ions which make us irritable, nervous and tired. And this is reflected in how we sleep. Studies have shown that negative ions promote relaxation, whilst positive ions cause migraine and insomnia.

and country ions… To breathe in negative ions, it is of course best to be in the open air in the countryside, in the mountains or by the sea. But another alternative is to put an air ionizer in your bedroom. An air ionizer is a small, silent electrical device that produces negative ions whilst you sleep. Put the appliance near your bed, because it can diffuse negative ions up to a distance of only 1.5 m (5 ft).

● ● ● DID YOU KNOW?

> Negative ions are produced naturally due to the effect of ionizing rays (such as solar rays or the soil's radioactivity) on the oxygen in the air. They also occur as a result of the disintegration of water droplets in the atmosphere (waterfalls and waves, for example).

KEY FACTS

* Studies show that negative ions help promote sleep.

* To breathe in enough negative ions, you need to go walking in the countryside or buy yourself an ionizer.

24 eat royal jelly

Royal jelly is made by worker bees to feed their larvae and the queen bee. Extremely rich in B-group vitamins and in essential minerals, this is the food of relaxation and good sleep.

Extremely nutritious: worker bees secrete royal jelly between the sixth and the twelfth day of their lives. They feed this glossy, gelatinous and slightly sweet product to the larvae for the first three days of their development. This unique food is all they need to multiply their weight a thousand times.

Exceptionally rich: royal jelly is a concentrate of nutrients essential to our health. It contains B-group vitamins, antibiotics, minerals including copper, calcium, iron, phosphorus, silicon and sulphur, as well as essential amino acids. Its extraordinary richness is thought to make it particularly good for physical and nervous relaxation. A course of royal jelly may recharge the batteries, dispel fatigue, improve cell renewal and promote mental and nervous well-being, all wonderful weapons in the battle against insomnia.

● ● ● DID YOU KNOW?

> It's advisable to take royal jelly for twenty-one days at each change of season. Royal jelly is available in phials, capsules or small pots. Whichever way you take it, the prescribed dose is 200 to 300 mg each morning before breakfast.

KEY FACTS

* Royal jelly is the food produced by worker bees for their larvae and the queen bee.

* It is extremely rich in B-group vitamins, minerals and amino acids.

* Royal jelly is thought to dispel tiredness and improve mental and nervous well-being.

25

give autogenic training a try

Relaxing the body and the mind at the same time – that is the basic principle of all relaxation methods. Autogenic training enables you to attain this state of total calm. Practise this simple technique, which anyone can do, every day to help you sleep better.

Calm, comfort and perseverance

Developed by the German physician, Johannes Schultz (1884-1970) at the beginning of the twentieth century, autogenic training is a perfect way of relaxing to regain sleep. It helps you banish black thoughts, relax the body and channel emotional excesses. For Schultz, the person is a physical and mental unity. He believed that these two levels of existence were inextricably linked, which was a novel idea for the time. To practise autogenic training, all you need is a quiet place, a comfortable position and a little perseverance. Practise three times a day for about ten minutes.

Six exercises for improving sleep

Lie down in a quiet, dark place. There are six exercises to a sequence. Each time, you must concentrate on the sensation and fix it by saying to yourself one of the following key phrases or mantras:

① **'I am totally calm.'**
② **'I can feel my body becoming heavy.'** Try to feel this heaviness in your shoulders, your arms, your body and your legs.
③ **'My body is warm.'** Feel this warmth throughout your body as in the previous exercise.
④ **'I can feel my heart beating calmly.'** Notice the pulsing action of your heart.
⑤ **'I can feel my breathing.'** Feel your lungs as they rise and fall with each breath you take.
⑥ **'I can feel the coolness on my forehead.'** Feel this cool breath as it passes over your forehead.
Then move your legs slightly, stretch and breathe in deeply. You can open your eyes to come back to reality or keep them shut to drift into sleep.

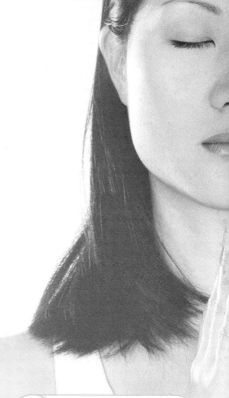

 KEY FACTS

* Autogenic training is both a simple and practical technique for relaxation.

* Its six exercises help you to get to sleep quickly.

* After a time, you can use it whenever you want to relax and calm yourself, without anyone noticing.

26

discover flower power

Concentrated flower essences can calm our emotional excesses and harmonize the balance of our soul. They are invaluable at times when we are losing sleep due to stress, an accumulation of worries or a major annoyance.

The strong soul of flowers

To produce an essence, the flower is picked at first light, placed in a bowl of pure water and then left exposed to the sun's rays. When the flower has withered, the water, which has been enriched by the flower's 'vibrations', is filtered and mixed with the same quantity of alcohol to stabilize it. Flower essences thus obtained are an effective way of treating psychological and emotional imbalances,

● ● ● DID YOU KNOW?

> The English physician, Dr Edward Bach (1886–1936), who practised at the beginning of the twentieth century, became convinced that the key to health could be found not in the human body, but in its soul. 'What we call illness is the terminal state of a much deeper disorder,' he wrote. His research led him to look at flowers, the final stage of the plant's development, which contain all the plant's vitality. He made dilutions from them and established relationships between the flowers and the conditions of the soul. This is how flower essences first came into being.

such as depression, aggression, timidity, lack of self-confidence and distress, and the sleeping problems they produce.

Essences come in dropper bottles. Prepare your diluted essence each morning for the whole day by adding two drops of pure essence to a glass of spring water, and take one teaspoonful four times a day between meals.

Five flower essences that 'work'

Identify the state you feel you are in and choose your essence accordingly:

- **You are always having to deal with the same problems, yet do not learn from experience:** take chestnut bud to increase your ability to adapt.
- **You are a pessimist, subject to doubt; you mull over problems in your head until you are exhausted:** take gentian to maintain your self-confidence, perseverance and willpower.
- **You are indecisive, you question everything:** take annual knawel (*Scleranthus annuus*) to help you keep a hold on reality.
- **You are mentally tired:** take hornbeam to give you more energy and enthusiasm.
- **You have just suffered a deep shock:** take Star of Bethlehem to free you from present and past stresses.

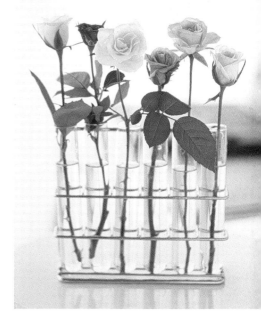

KEY FACTS

* Flower essences are concentrated extracts of flowers.

* They bring the states of the soul into harmony.

* They relieve insomnia due to emotional troubles.

27 try a light cure

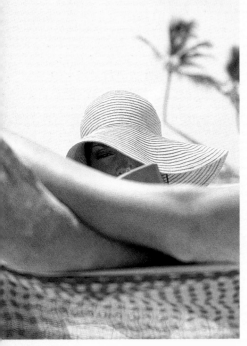

Insomnia can sometimes be due to winter depression or **SAD (Seasonal Affective Disorder)**. Lack of light causes some people to become sad, weighed down and exhausted. Their sleep is disturbed, only to return to normal once the better weather arrives. One solution is light therapy.

> According to this study, light therapy is best used as a preventative method: a dozen sessions in autumn, when the first indications appear, will prevent the problems from becoming entrenched.

● ● ● DID YOU KNOW?

> According to a Japanese study, light therapy relieves up to 48% of cases of seasonal depression and the insomnia that goes with it.

It's going to be a long, hard winter

In winter, when the days are shorter, some people are affected by a depression that can manifest itself either as hypersomnia (they are always sleepy) or alternatively as insomnia (they cannot sleep). When the better weather arrives, sleep returns to its normal pattern … until the following winter.

These problems are due to disturbances to the biological rhythms affected by light. The light rays filtered by the retina do not only help us to see clearly, they penetrate our brain where they stimulate the production of certain neuro-hormones, especially melatonin. When we produce too little of these hormones, an imbalance is created in the brain which leads to disturbed sleep.

Let there be light!

The treatment is simple: at specific times, the patient is exposed to an extremely intense light (between 2,500 and 10,000 lux depending on the case) for a period that can range from half-an-hour to six hours a day. The treatment is carried out on a daily basis and can continue for up to three weeks.

Light therapy is carried out either in a hospital environment or in some psychiatric practices. You can also buy special lamps that you can use in the comfort of your own home.

KEY FACTS

* Some types of insomnia are due to seasonal depression.

* In winter, the lack of light can disturb the biochemical balance of the brain.

* Light therapy involves exposing the patient to a 'bath' of light.

* The treatment is administered in a hospital environment or in psychiatric practices.

* You can also buy special lamps that you can use in the comfort of your own home.

28

choose the right colours for you

Colours have an effect on our health, our behaviour and the balance of our lives. Red is a stimulating colour whereas blue is relaxing. Through feng shui the Chinese have refined the art of colour in the home.

Warm and cold tones

In the past red was used in the room in which children suffering from measles, in the hope that they would recover more quickly. A purple pillowcase was thought to help insomniacs sleep better. It is a fact that colours can influence our behaviour. Cold colours, such as blue or purple, calm us down. Warm tones, such as red or orange, are stimulants and excite us.

● ● ● DID YOU KNOW?

> Colours do not exist; by that is meant that they do not have a material existence.

> They are in fact electromagnetic waves of different lengths and our brain translates them into sensations of colour.

The colours of energy

According to the principles of feng shui, colours can accelerate or slow down the circulation of energy in the home, depending on the fundamental layout of the room. Colours are selected according to the way your room faces and they slow down the energy in the walls, curtains and carpets.

- **North:** green (light or dark) and blue
- **Northeast:** pink, white and grey
- **West to southwest:** shades of purple to light mauve
- **South:** white, pale yellow and light brown shades
- **Southwest:** white, grey and pink
- **West to northwest:** cream and off-white

The colour yellow is linked symbolically to the element of Earth and, as such, it represents the 'centre' and with it 'harmony'. You can use it in any room, regardless of the direction it faces, without interrupting the flow of vital energy.

> That is why certain intermediary colours are difficult to define. Turquoise is interpreted as blue by one person and green by another. It is the same with violet, thought by some to be mauve and others pink.

KEY FACTS

* Traditionally bedrooms are decorated in cold, relaxing colours, notably blue or green.

* According to the principles of feng shui, colours are selected according to the way the room faces.

* You need to channel the circulation of energy to improve sleep.

29 remove electrical appliances

Bedrooms are often full of electrical appliances that pollute the environment by emitting waves, even when switched off.

Poor, defenceless sleepers! When we sleep, our bodies lose 70% of their defences against external influences. This makes us especially sensitive to electromagnetic radiation, emitted by such appliances as televisions, computers and radio alarms, often found in bedrooms. In the same way as an aerial, the human body picks up all these signals. If there are too many of them, they end up disturbing the body's cells. They affect our whole sense of balance, and the quality of our sleep suffers accordingly.

Emergency measures:
• Avoid placing electrical appliances near your bed, particularly if you have a mesh-strung divan base or metal bedstead.
• If you must have electric appliances in the bedroom, make sure you disconnect them when they are not in use.
• Remember to cover screens (e.g. television, computer) with a silk cloth. This deadens the radiation emitted when the appliances are switched off. The screen actually continues to emit radiation for several minutes after the appliance has been disconnected.

● ● ● DID YOU KNOW?

> It's best to avoid sleeping with your head against a load-bearing wall because the wall transmits electromagnetic pollution from one floor to another.

KEY FACTS

∗ Electrical appliances, such as radio-alarms, televisions and computers, disturb sleep.

∗ Avoid putting these appliances in the bedroom.

30 understand the role of magnesium

Magnesium is the Number 1 nutrient for the nervous system. Without it, we become tense, anxious and above all unable to sleep. To ensure we get enough magnesium, it is essential to eat foods such as dried fruit and chocolate and to take a magnesium cure regularly.

Long live chocolate! A lack of magnesium can lead to trembling, cramp, tetany attacks, irritability and most especially insomnia. Magnesium occurs naturally in dried fruit, pulses, chocolate and wholemeal bread.

500 mg to 1 g per day: The generally recommended daily dose for an adult is about 400 mg but if you are stressed, you will need considerably more. Some medicines, such as antibiotics, increase the requirement still further. To regain sleep when you are tense and anxious, take 500 mg of magnesium (together with 250 mg calcium) at bedtime. You can also take a magnesium cure for three to four weeks every three months. Vitamin B6 helps the body to assimilate the magnesium which is contraindicated in the case of renal insufficiency.

● ● ● DID YOU KNOW?

> Excessive consumption of refined sugar 'eats up' our reserves of magnesium as refined sugar burns up our stores of nutrients that the body turns into energy. If you enjoy your food too much, if you tend to eat sweet things to ease your tensions away, it's advisable to take magnesium supplements.

KEY FACTS

* Magnesium may play a role in the correct transmission of nerve impulses.

* A supplement of between 500 mg to 1 g of magnesium per day can improve sleep.

31 put your worries in context

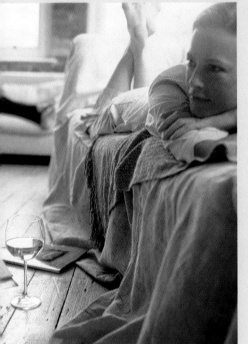

During periods of extreme stress, our thoughts often race around in our heads. It is impossible to make them stop at the end of the day in order to get a refreshing night's sleep. If you want to sleep well, however, you really must have a calm mind.

> According to him, most of the time we function on the basis of wrong thoughts and it is these thoughts that make us suffer, not reality. To get better, we must drive the wrong thoughts out and replace them with healthy thoughts.

When the gods are against us …

A baby who passes away with barely a cry; a child who is always getting into trouble at school; a loved-one suffering a terrible illness… sometimes the gods seem to be against us. The first time this happens, we manage to cope with the situation using reflection, evaluation and control. But if the distress accumulates or if it persists without our being able to find a solution, we break down, and that is exactly when sleep decides to elude us. There is only one way of regaining it: we have to make peace with our thoughts and thus with ourselves.

Stand back

When we are unable to control our environment, it is useless to exhaust ourselves trying to change it. But there is always one thing that we can change: ourselves. Our life is built up on the basis of received ideas inherited from childhood, education, society. Over the years we have absorbed these ideas without noticing it. Periods of crisis are the perfect times for us to take stock of our real desires, our fundamental aspirations:

• What do I really expect of life?
• What are my priorities?
• What aims would I like to achieve?
• What have I given up since my adolescence?
• How can I achieve these objectives?

It's not always as simple as that, but it is sometimes essential if we are to regain serenity, inner balance and quality natural sleep.

KEY FACTS

∗ At times of crisis and stress, we find it difficult to calm our thoughts when we are trying to get to sleep.

∗ This is the ideal moment to determine what is really important for us and what is not.

∗ We can learn the ability to have healthy thoughts.

> Healthy thoughts are based on objective facts; they help us protect our life and our health; they enable us to achieve our aims and to avoid conflicts in relationships and help us deal with our emotions.

32

practise meditation

One meaning of meditation is to take time to contemplate a thought until you have considered it from all aspects. In Eastern thinking, however, it means silencing the mind, emptying it of all its contents to find peace. It is a difficult exercise but can be very useful when trying to regain sleep.

Try meditation

Zen is a philosophy derived from Buddhism that developed in Japan. Minimalist in form, it centres round a posture: silent sitting, also called Zazen. Zen masters have a habit of saying that there is no point talking about it, just do it. Experiments have shown that practising Zazen puts the cortex (the seat of conscious thought) at rest, whilst the limbic brain (the seat of the emotions) remains

● ● ● DID YOU KNOW?

> Zazen can be practised in a group at a Zen centre (dojo) under a master who leads the session and corrects posture.

> You can also take part in seminars lasting several days.

active. When meditating the blood flow increases, thereby improving the oxygenation of the cells. The brain waves slow down and this sees the start of a period of intense relaxation, which encourages sleep.

Practising Zazen

All you have to do is get yourself a small, hard, circular cushion (zafu) and sit on it in a quiet place about one metre (three feet) from a wall. With knees bent and legs crossed, place your right foot on top of your left thigh and draw your left foot back against the cushion. With your back very straight and chin down, imagine that you are pushing against the sky with the top of your head. Your hands should be at the level of your navel, with the left hand placed over the right and palms facing upwards. Half-close your eyes, fixing your gaze at the foot of the wall in front of you.

Now all you have to do is to breathe whilst concentrating on your out-breath which must be long, slow and very deep. Watch your thoughts slip away like clouds in the sky but do not try to catch them. It is difficult to start with. With practise, the thoughts become fewer and fewer, and less and less obsessive.

> Once you have acquired the correct posture, you can also practise Zazen on your own at home, on the beach, in the wood … the important thing is to meditate regularly.

KEY FACTS

* Zen philosophy is not learnt, it is practised.

* Zazen is the seated meditation posture of Zen Buddhism.

* This practice induces a sense of calm and relaxation that encourages sound sleep.

* You can practise it either on your own or in a group.

33

keep laughing

On average, our grandparents spent almost 20 minutes a day laughing. Today, laughter accounts for only 5 minutes of our day. And yet it is a powerful tool for physical, nervous and mental relaxation, perfect for falling asleep feeling calm and care-free.

A physiological phenomenon

Laughter is a set of small, spasmodic out-breaths produced by involuntary contractions of the diaphragm. Some muscles are set in motion, whilst others relax. The sudden expulsion of breath produces the characteristic noises of laughter. When all's said and done, there is nothing very funny about the physiological definition of laughter!

● ● ● DID YOU KNOW?

> As far back as Classical times, the Roman physician, Galen, affirmed that 'cheerful women recover more quickly than miserable women.'

> In the thirteenth century, the French surgeon, Henri de Mondeville, advocated laughter as a therapy: 'The surgeon,' he said, 'will forbid his patient to feel anger, hatred and sadness.'

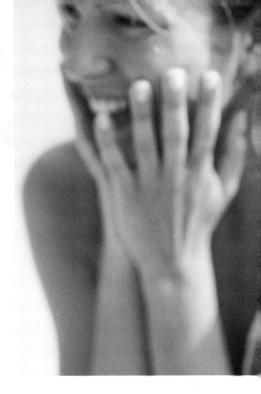

Laughter can be caused by an intellectual stimulus (such as a witty remark or a funny scene); a physical stimulus (such as tickling, inhalation of laughing gas); or an illness, such as schizophrenia.

The big clear-out

Whatever the cause, the least ripple of laughter and a real clear-out starts up in your body: you clean and air your respiratory tracts; you increase your secretion of saliva and gastric juices (thus improving the digestion); your stomach and intestines contract (thus improving evacuation of waste). The chemical exchanges within your brain also change: a surplus of endorphins reduces stress and soothes distress, nervousness and anxiety, all of which cheerfully helps re-establish healthy sleeping patterns. All you need now is to be blessed with an easy laugh!

> 'He will remind the patient that the body is fortified by means of joy and is weakened by sadness.'

KEY FACTS

* We are laughing less and less.

* Laughter improves the general functioning of the body and reduces nervousness, distress and anxiety.

* Laughter alters the chemistry of the brain, making it produce more endorphins.

34
control
your energy

According to traditional Chinese medicine, insomnia may be the result of an excess of energy in the heart meridian. A Qi Gong exercise can help to restore balance and encourage better sleep.

Energy and balance

Balance and health depend on our vital energy according to Chinese medicine. If energy circulates harmoniously, then all is well. Difficulty arises when it is interrupted, blocked, in deficit or excess. This energy travels along canals known as meridians. Insomnia can be triggered by too much energy in the heart meridian but, if it is dispersed properly, sleep can return.

Stretch your heart

Qi Gong is one of the therapeutic instruments in Chinese medicine. It involves the 'stretching' of the heart meridian in order to regulate the flow of energy.

① Stand upright, feet parallel and slightly apart, back nice and straight – bend your knees gently.

② Cross your arms in front of your chest, keeping your upper arms, wrists and fingers relaxed.

③ Raise your arms whilst keeping them bent, open them out and turn your palms upwards.

④ Uncross your arms above your head and then lower them to your sides. Return your arms to the chest position, palms facing upwards.

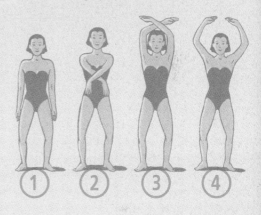

> Complete this exercise slowly, breathing deeply and trying to empty your mind. You can 'stretch' this meridian or energy channel every day in this manner in order to maintain the energy of the element of Fire, linked symbolically to the heart. It will help you sleep better and relieve headaches, anxiety and feelings of panic.

KEY FACTS

* In Chinese medicine, sleeping problems are attributed to poor circulation of energy in the body.

* Insomnia is due to an excess of energy in the heart meridian.

* Practise stretching the heart meridian to improve sleep.

35

massage
your wrists

Derived from traditional Chinese medicine, *do-in* has a beneficial effect on the circulation of vital energy in the body. It involves direct intervention, using the bare hands, on the acupuncture points.

A tool to promote health and balance

Less precise than acupuncture, *do-in* has the advantage that it can be practised at home, with family or friends – there is no need to go to a doctor's surgery. You can massage yourself or other people. It is a tool to promote health and well-being that anybody can acquire and use in their daily life.

Do-in tones the skin, activates circulation of the blood and lymph system and helps eliminate toxins; it regulates the activity of the neuro-vegetative nervous system, calms mental and emotional tensions, relieves pain, stimulates organ function and improves the functioning of the endocrine glands. It is an excellent way of combating insomnia.

A 'special sleep' session

This massage, to relieve tension and promote peaceful sleep, involves pressing firmly with the thumb on the two points on the wrists shown below and rotating the thumb in a clockwise, circular movement. The massage should be vigorous and firm but not painful.

• **The first point** is at the centre of the inside of the wrist, just at the base of the hand.
• **The second point** is situated two finger-widths behind the first point.

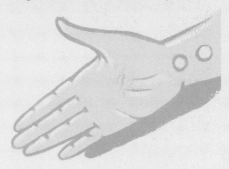

KEY FACTS

∗ By massaging the acupuncture points, *do-in* has a beneficial effect on the circulation of vital energy.

∗ The two points that have an effect on sleep are located on the inside of the wrists.

∗ *Do-in* can also be carried out on the whole body to relax, relieve tension and combat fatigue.

36

imagine the perfect sleep

Imagination to help the mind and the body: that is one way of defining visualization. By imagining the ideal scenario for falling asleep and waking up, you can relax your mind and body and capture the sleep that is eluding you.

As real as a real lemon

We all do visualization without realising it. Unfortunately, we use this technique in a negative way: we tend to imagine the worst to prepare ourselves for failure, to 'foresee' difficulties. If you want to benefit from the positive aspects of visualization, all you have to do is go into reverse. By imagining things in the most positive light possible, we can prepare ourselves to embrace success.

●●● DID YOU KNOW?

> The origins of visualization are lost in the mists of time. In primitive societies, rituals performed before major hunts included some positive visualization. People in the Far East practise it using meditation or concentration as part of their religious rites.

> Even prayer can be viewed from this angle: you focus on yourself and then you conjure up positive images to back up the plea.

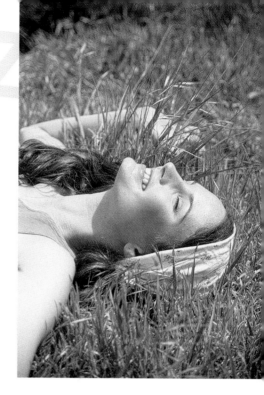

Our body reacts to these images as though they were really happening. Try it for yourself: shut your eyes and imagine a beautiful, bright yellow lemon. Then imagine yourself cutting it and biting into a quarter of it. The acidity pervades your mouth; the juice runs over your lips. Then what happens? You salivate! The simple act of imagining the lemon has produced the same effect (or nearly) as a real lemon. The same applies to all our biological functions.

Give free rein to your imagination

To fall asleep more quickly and sleep more peacefully and soundly, all you have to do is settle down comfortably in your bed, close your eyes, breathe deeply and imagine the perfect place to sleep: a beach lulled by the lapping of the waves, a hammock strung between two pine trees, a meadow scattered with wildflowers, a four-poster bed. Your imagination need know no bounds. The more the sounds, smells and colours of the scene find echoes in your mind, the more effective the visualization will be. It's up to you to imagine how things proceed, until you fall asleep.

KEY FACTS

* We all visualize things without knowing it, but in a negative way.

* To pave the way for success, all you have to do is to visualize positive images.

* Visualize yourself in an ideal place and imagine the sleep that you achieve.

37

make love!

Making love in the evening is an excellent way to prepare yourself for sleep. After the tension of desire and the explosion of pleasure, comes a natural relaxation that helps you to sleep. Provided, of course, that there are no sexual difficulties in the relationship.

The endorphin story

There is a therapeutic dimension to sensual pleasure. Orgasm is a source of health, even of healing. Throughout the sexual act, our body secretes substances that promote pleasure, relaxation and calm. These include endorphins: natural hormones, related to morphine, that cause comparable effects (euphoria, calm, disappearance of tensions and pain). Produced in the brain, these

● ● ● DID YOU KNOW?

> The sense of touch lies at the very heart of sexual pleasure and the subsequent relaxation that promotes sleep.

> Sexual abandon is a form of regression, where we rediscover the sensations of early childhood with caresses, strokes and tender touches.

hormones spread throughout the body, relaxing the muscles, regulating the nervous system, improving circulation of the blood and increasing respiratory capacity. All of which are preconditions for sound sleep.

Orgasm at all costs

To make the most of these benefits, it is important that sex is also calm and care-free. In men, it is erection problems that can sometimes cause a block. In women, it's the quest for orgasm at all costs that often causes difficulties. If you experience such problems, try to resolve them first by consulting a sexologist or a psychologist, who will help you to take the time to understand your body anew and to discover the origin of your blocks. That way, you will be able to start making love again at night, before gently slipping from sensual pleasure into sleep.

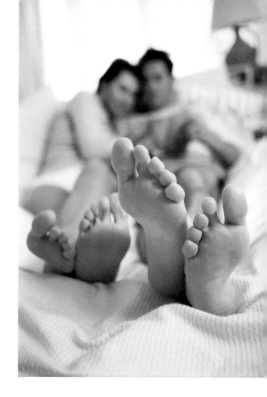

> These actions make us feel safe, calm and relaxed. Our adult 'shell' gradually gives way to tenderness. A sure way to get to sleep.

 KEY FACTS

* Making love helps our bodies secrete the pleasure hormones, especially endorphins.

* Good sex has a regulating effect on the entire body.

* If you have sexual difficulties, do not hesitate to seek the advice of an expert.

38

enjoy a shoulder massage

Our skin is an important sensory organ. When massaged with relaxing essential oils, it transmits messages to us that help us relax and fall asleep. Simple and easy to do, this shoulder massage will help you fall asleep.

Millions of sensors

Our skin is not just an envelope: it is a whole parcel of gifts. It conceals millions of sensors which give us information about the outside world (heat and humidity, for example) and transmit messages to us, both positive and negative (relaxation and serenity, but also discomfort and pain). Whatever the technique applied, massage uses the skin as a vehicle to help us relax our muscles and calm our mental state.

To prepare yourself for sleep, ask someone close to you – your partner, friend or child – to give you a shoulder massage.

Lavender, sweet orange and jasmine

Prepare your massage oil by mixing together 200 ml (6½ fl oz) of apricot or jojoba oil with 20 drops of a mixture of relaxing, fragrant essential oils (such as lavender, sweet orange, jasmine or ylang ylang). Pour a tablespoonful of this oil into a saucer; then proceed as follows:

• First massage the base of the skull and the shoulders on each side of the nape of the neck.

• Massage the shoulders; then move down along the arms to the elbows, using small, circular movements.

• Work back up towards the nape of the neck.

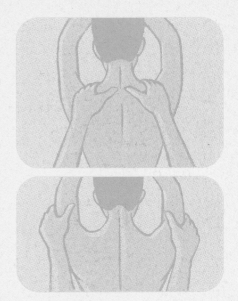

• Finally, repeat the whole sequence about ten times.

KEY FACTS

∗ The skin contains millions of sensors.

∗ Massage transmits calming and relaxing messages via these sensors.

∗ This shoulder massage helps you prepare for sleep.

∗ Use essential oils such as lavender, sweet orange, jasmine and ylang ylang.

The monsters that inhabited our childhood nights sometimes come back to haunt us in times of stress, making us experience our terrors of yesteryear anew, waking us during the night and preventing us from getting back to sleep. Homeopathy can help us stamp them out.

39

say goodbye to your nightmares

Unfinished images

Nightmares are no respecters of age. These frightening and sometimes gory nocturnal images can suddenly appear at any stage in life. They are an expression of the deep anxieties that sweep through the limbo of our subconscious, taking advantage of the fact that our minds are more vulnerable when we sleep. To banish these intruders forever sometimes requires a visit to a specialist.

●●● DID YOU KNOW?

> According to the principle of similitude, on which homeopathy is based, a substance administered in a tiny dose remedies the effects that it produces if given in a large dose to a healthy person.

> For example, peeling onions makes the eyes water and the nose tickle. Onion dilution (*Allium cepa*) treats colds characterized by a runny nose and watery, stinging eyes.

However, if it's just a matter of making them back off a bit so that you can regain more peaceful sleep, then homeopathy is an alternative option.

Dreams of death, fire and blood

Depending on the content of the images that regularly return in your nightmares, a homeopathic doctor will prescribe a specific medication for you. Here are a few examples:
• Dreams involving death: *Lachesis mutus; Calcarea carbonica.*
• Dreams involving ferocious animals: *Argentum nitricum; Opium.*
• Dreams involving blood or bleeding: *Phosphorus.*
• Dreams involving falling or an accident: *Arnica montana, Lycopodium.*
• Dreams involving feelings of helplessness: *Rhus toxidodendron.*
These medicines should be taken in doses of 9 C (5 grains) at night before going to bed).

> In the same way, certain substances produce specific dreams which their dilutions can make disappear.

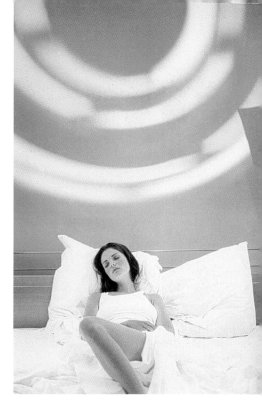

KEY FACTS

* Nightmares can strike at any age.

* To discover what nightmares mean, we need to explore our subconscious.

* Suitable homeopathic medicines can calm distressing nights.

40 manage your time properly

Time is a great enemy of sleep. The excessive stress of our working day sometimes steals from us those precious hours that bring us rest. And yet, if we learn to manage it properly, time can become a night-time ally.

Friend or foe? Time passes at a different rhythm, depending on whether we are enduring it or enjoying it, leaving us more or less tired and exhausted at the end of the day. If you're looking for a refreshing night's sleep, enjoyment is your best option.

The ground rules:
• Set yourself specific and realistic goals for the day.
• Draw up a list of your tasks for the day and tick them off as you achieve them.
• Respect your body's natural rhythm: for example, don't put yourself down for sport first thing in the afternoon if you tend to feel shattered then.
• Whatever your agenda, make sure you always keep a little time free for pleasure. Dare to say no.

● ● ● DID YOU KNOW?

> It is often the quest for perfection that makes us manage our time badly. We cannot be perfect professionals, impeccable parents and ideal partners all at once. To prevent ourselves from being overburdened, we have got to learn to be tolerant towards ourselves and to accept help.

KEY FACTS

* Time that flies is an enemy, while well-managed time is an ally.

* Set yourself specific goals and respect your body's natural rhythm.

* Set aside time for yourself and accept help.

case study

I learned to sleep by practising meditation.

'All these stories make me smile. For me, there was a spiritual aspect to meditation and I'm not much of a believer. However, for several years I had gone through bad patches, as far as sleep was concerned, during periods of stress at work. I used to lose sleep by dint of turning over my problems again and again in my mind. And at night, when you can't sleep, the smallest problem assumes massive proportions, far removed from reality. In the morning, things return to their normal size, problems become manageable again. But, the next evening, it starts all over again and being aware of this makes no difference. I ended up by acting on the advice of a friend, who took me to a dojo to learn how to meditate. I really got into it. The first time, I felt that my thoughts were buzzing around in my head like flies; I wished I'd had a "thought-killer spray" to get rid of them all. It was several months before I really started to be able to control the flow of thoughts in my mind. And that was the end of my insomnia. I meditate for 15 minutes each morning, and sometimes in the evening if I feel tense. Meditation has changed my life!'

41 >>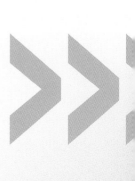

>> **When sleep just won't come,** your health can really start to deteriorate.

>>>> Initially, you think you are getting used to the tiredness and you draw on newly discovered inner reserves. But after many months of this, you end up quietly sinking into a sort of physical and mental exhaustion. **You have got to do something about it.**

>>>>>> Any method is good if it **helps solve the problem.** Whether it's following basic rules for a healthy lifestyle, selective techniques or some more powerful therapies, all these can help avoid the systematic use of chemical sleeping pills as far as possible.

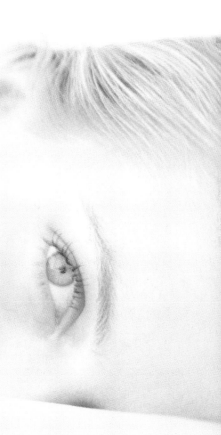

60
TIPS

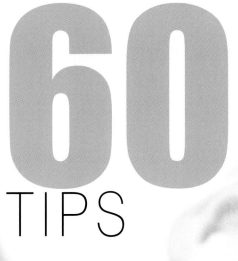

41 analyze your insomnia

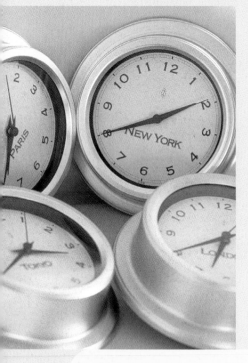

In order to combat long-term insomnia, it is important to work out the causes, identify the circumstances that provoke it and understand the way your body works and reacts. It is time to do a self-assessment.

early or to sleep fitfully. It is vital to take these symptoms into account as they can be tackled by different treatments – natural plant and homeopathic remedies, acupuncture etc.

Your worst nights – a guide to surviving them

Insomnia is defined as difficulty in experiencing qualitative or quantitative sleep. It embraces a number of different problems with diverse causes and many different manifestations. In order to get to the bottom of your problem, you need to understand more about insomnia, and the only way to do this is to monitor it. Take out your notebook (see pages 12-13) and keep a record of your worst nights' sleep, noting what you ate, what you did the day before, whom you met, what the temperature was and the level of humidity. You will soon be able to identify the elements that play a part in your lack of sleep.

Digestion, circulation, anxiety

These causes of insomnia can be treated differently.
• **Digestive:** some people sleep badly when their digestive system is overworked, slow and heavy.

• **Circulatory:** poor circulation can cause disruption to your sleeping pattern (heavy legs, pain, oedema)
• **Psychological:** worrying about a problem can cause sleep deprivation. Moving or taking a journey can make it harder to sleep, due to the strange surroundings.

KEY FACTS

* Understand more about insomnia and you will start to solve it.

* Insomnia can be due to digestive, circulatory or psychological problems.

* Difficulty getting to sleep, awakening too early or sleeping fitfully – all these are forms of insomnia.

> Spend time understanding your insomnia in order to treat it properly

42

reduce your intake of sleeping tablets

More and more people are turning to psychotropic drugs that affect the mind. Sleeping tablets, tranquilizers or narcotics, however, are all very addictive and their side effects are by no means slight.

Chemistry and sickness of the soul

There is no chemical that cures sicknesses of the soul. Yet it is often in moments of psychological, relational or emotional crisis that people turn to psychotropic drugs. Although they then experience a rapid improvement, this is short-lived, their dose is therefore increased and they quickly become addicted. If you want to be shot of them altogether, you really must come off them gradually. If you stop taking the medication too suddenly, the symptoms return even more forcefully than before. If you have been taking sleeping tables every day for several months, seek your doctor's advice but if you have been taking them just every now and again or for less than a month, you can try to reduce the dose yourself.

Planned withdrawal

There are three stages to the withdrawal process:

• **Stage 1:** reduce the dose of your medicines by half and supplement with the appropriate homeopathic or herbal remedies for your particular case.

• **Stage 2:** after three weeks, depending on the case, reduce your dose by half again whilst continuing to use natural remedies.

• **Stage 3:** after a further three weeks, stop using your medicines totally and continue with your homeopathic or herbal remedies.

You can then gradually start to reduce your doses of herbal or homeopathic pills to suit you and then take them less frequently until you can stop altogether.

●●● DID YOU KNOW?

> Some doctors use the placebo effect to wean their patients off drugs. You can try the bread pellet method for yourself. Make seven bread pellets (one per day for one week) and hide a sleeping tablet in six of them. Mix them up so that you do not know which is the empty pellet. Take one each night for a week. For the second week, place a sleeping tablet in only five of the pellets and so on. The fact that you don't know which nights you are actually taking the medicine means that you will not be able to 'anticipate' the return of insomnia.

KEY FACTS

∗ More and more people are turning to psychotropic drugs.

∗ These medicines can cause pharmacological addiction.

∗ Sleep studies have shown that subjects consistently underestimate how much they have actually slept.

What type of homeopathy is right for you? See if you can spot yourself in this gallery of portraits. If you find several similarities, all you have to do is take the corresponding medicine to gently relieve your insomnia.

43

learn how homeopathy can help you

Rigorous experiments

When he perfected homeopathy, Samuel Hahnemann (1755-1843) tested all the substances in the pharmacopoeia of the time (plants, animal and mineral products) on himself, his close friends and his family to note the effects they produced. By virtue of the principle of similitude, minute dilutions of these substances cured all these effects.

As some effects were physical and others were emotional or behavioural,

● ● ● D I D   Y O U   K N O W ?

> There are many more homeopathic remedies, and more powerful ones at that, than those that we have just touched on.

> If you think you recognize yourself in this outline, try taking a 9 C dose of the appropriate medicine, 3 grains every morning and night, for a month.

Hahnemann was soon able to spot identifiable 'types' that corresponded with the major remedies. We never conform completely to one of these types. But if we recognize ourselves, even partially, in one of these types, we have everything to gain from taking the corresponding medicine. It will relieve our excesses and re-establish disrupted equilibrium, including problems with sleeping.

A few portraits

- *Argentum nitricum:* You are always in a hurry, irritable and anxious. You do not like crowds, large open spaces or high places. You console yourself by eating sweet things, especially chocolate.
- *Arsenicum album:* You are frightened of death and illness. An obsessive, you check that you have locked the door ten times before going out. You feel the cold.

> If you see no improvement, consult a homeopathic doctor who will be able to refine the treatment to suit you.

- *Gelsemium sempervirens:* A nervous wreck! Whenever you speak in public or take an exam, you babble helplessly or your mind goes blank.
- *Ignatia amara:* You are ultra-sensitive to paradoxical reactions. You are always overworked and end up making more and more blunders as you act in haste.
- *Natrum muriaticum:* At the slightest shock to the system, you lose weight as well as sleep, even though you usually enjoy your food, especially savoury dishes.
- *Nux vomica:* You wake at about three o'clock in the morning and don't get to sleep again until just before the alarm clock goes off. You are quick-tempered and do not like to be thwarted.

KEY FACTS

* Homeopathic trials made it possible to list 'types' corresponding to major remedies.

* If you recognize yourself in one of these portraits, take the appropriate medicine. It will moderate your excesses and re-establish your disrupted equilibrium.

44 discover the power of the micro-dose

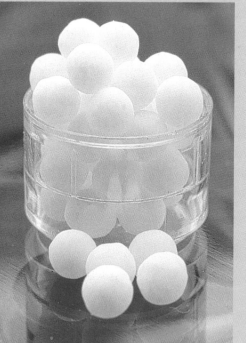

In addition to the basic medicine, homeopathic remedies have 'crisis' medicine aimed at combating very precise symptoms. Micro-doses do not treat an illness but the whole. Sleep can be treated in this way.

> Children can be treated with specific homeopathic remedies. *Chamomilla*, for example, relieves babies born with colic.

> *Causticum* helps anxious children terrified by the dark to sleep.
> *Pulsatilla* is given to children with separation anxiety, unable to sleep alone for fear of abandonment.

Hot or cold, sweet or savoury?

Homeopathy focuses on the way symptoms present. That is why a homeopathic doctor will often ask questions that appear to be unconnected to the condition, such as what you like to eat, what you dream about, if you can tolerate extremes of heat or cold, what you most fear. This information helps the doctor to determine the most appropriate medication for you as an individual. Self-treatment with homeopathic medicine is therefore not easy, since objective assessment of one's self is difficult.

Research a remedy

The medicines listed here can be taken to help fight insomnia. Assess which one seems most appropriate for you and take 3 pills morning and night. If you do not achieve the desired result after two to three weeks, consult a homeopathic doctor and he or she will be able to refine the treatment and prescribe appropriate solutions and dosage.
• You cannot get to sleep, you ache all over and feel stiff: *Arnica*.
• Your emotions are running so high you cannot sleep: *Ignatia*.
• You feel over-excited and confused as if you have drunk too much coffee: *Cafea*.

• You are in a bad mood, tired out by too much thinking: *Kalium phosphoricum*.
• You stop being sleepy as soon as you go to bed: *Hyoscyamus*.
• Fear of the dark and nightmares is preventing sleep: *Stramonium*.
• You wake up at 4am with a feeling of indigestion or breathing difficulties: *Kalium carbonicum*.
• You wake up soon after falling asleep without being able to go back to sleep: *Belladonna*.

KEY FACTS

* Homeopathic medicine targets the specific symptoms of the individual patient.

* It is often difficult to find the appropriate remedy for one's self; it's best to consult a doctor .

* Certain homeopathic remedies can be used to treat children with sleeping problems.

45

consult a relaxation therapist

A bridge between East and West, this technique borrows from Zen, yoga, hypnosis and visualization. The relaxation therapist provides you with an effective skill that you can use on your own to make your nights even better than your days.

Images and keywords

This method was perfected by a Spanish psychiatrist, Alfonso Caycedo, in the Sixties. Inspired by oriental techniques, such as Zen and yoga, and western techniques, such as hypnosis, it uses a special state of consciousness, half-way between wakefulness and sleep, to evoke images and keywords that help attain a state of deep physical and mental relaxation.

Journey to the centre of yourself

Initially, relaxation therapy is practised with a therapist. During an initial discussion, the therapist will explore with you the modalities and origins of your insomnia. After that, the two of you will choose the elements of the guided course that make up the session.

There you are, comfortably lying down. The relaxation therapist asks you to breathe deeply with your eyes closed and then to relax your muscles one by one. Once you have reached 'the relaxed state', the therapist will guide you along a personal journey that you will have to repeat each evening at home. Some relaxation therapists make personalized accompanying cassettes to help the client at home. The session finishes with a discussion of how things have progressed. Four or five sessions are usually all you need to put a stop to stress-induced insomnia.

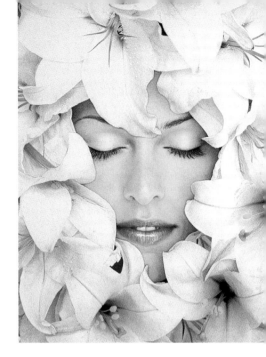

> It does not matter where you choose, just as long as it is a place where you feel good. You will retreat to your chosen place each evening to go to sleep.

KEY FACTS

* Falling between hypnosis and yoga, relaxation therapy is a method of guided relaxation that helps combat insomnia.

* Initially, it is practised under the guidance of a therapist, then at home on your own.

* Create a perfect space within yourself where you go each evening to fall asleep.

46

circulate your energy

To circulate the vital energy, which leads to insomnia if blocked, Taoist tradition suggests you 'massage' your organs. This is a simple and effective technique to calm the heart energy and invigorate that of the lungs so that you can regain sleep.

Manipulation and visualization

Taoist tradition teaches specific therapeutic massages that form the basis of Chinese medicine. This tradition is taught rigorously in Chinese schools and hospitals. Without going into too much detail, give 'organ massage' a try. Halfway between manipulation and visualization, these exercises help control the flow of energy in one of the five principal organs: the liver, the heart, the spleen, the lungs or the kidneys.

According to Chinese medicine, insomnia is usually caused by excess energy in the heart meridian. Massaging this organ will help drain this excess energy away.

A beneficial flow of energy

• First, place your hands flat, one on top of the other, at the top of your abdomen just where the sternum begins (see diagram 1). Close your eyes and start to breathe deeply.

• Imagine a flow of energy emanating from your hands, entering your body and flowing towards your heart.

• Feel the energy as it spreads out across your chest and then surrounds your heart itself.

• Breathe deeply for a few minutes, visualizing the organ that taps this energy to restore itself.

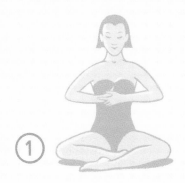

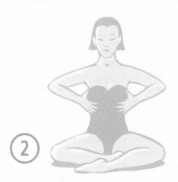

● ● ●   DID YOU KNOW?

> According to Chinese medicine, some types of insomnia can also be caused by a lack of energy in the lung meridian. To remedy this situation, you can do the same exercise, but this time placing your hands flat at the level of the lungs (see diagram 2), one on each side of the rib cage.

KEY FACTS

∗ Taoist tradition teaches a series of 'organ massages'.

∗ Halfway between manipulation and visualization, organ massage involves sending energy to the organs to revive them.

∗ Heart energy and, less frequently, lung energy cause insomnia.

47 trust in acupuncture

Acupuncture is the most invasive and most powerful therapy in Chinese medicine and involves inserting needles into the acupuncture points to control the energy flows.

Sleep points: acupuncture is a particularly effective way of re-establishing balance in the nervous system, which often has a rough time due to the stresses and emotional strains of modern living. That is why this therapy can treat stress-induced insomnia, even if it is a long-standing problem that has proved resistant to other treatments. And what's more, certain specific points act straight away by inducing sleep, although only a qualified acupuncturist will know where to find them.

Visit a therapist: acupuncture does not use any medicinal substances. It therefore involves no toxins at all. However, some people are put off by even the sight of a needle. If that is the case with you, don't force yourself; just go to a different type of therapist. If you are not put off by the needles, you can consult an acupuncturist who will know how to figure out your problem using the Chinese energy principles. You must go to a qualified acupuncturist for acupuncture treatments.

● ● ● D I D   Y O U   K N O W ?

> To avoid any risk of contamination, acupuncture therapists generally use sterile, single-use needles which are discarded after use. They can also 'heat' the points using a burning artemisia or moxa cone.

K E Y   F A C T S

* Certain specific acupuncture points induce sleep immediately.

* It is essential to consult an acupuncturist as this treatment cannot be done at home.

48 understand hormone treatment

Our sleep is partly governed by the subtle play of hormones. Certain slight imbalances can disturb our sleep.

The ravages of age: difficulties sleeping often appear with age because the endocrine glands, like the other tissues in the body, are subject to ageing, making them less active.

The sleep hormones:
• **Melatonin:** accelerates the falling asleep stage by slowing down the heart rate and reducing blood pressure. It prolongs the periods of paradoxical and deep sleep.
• **Sex hormones:** progesterone and oestrogens in women, testosterone in men, improve the quality of sleep.
• **Growth hormone:** this makes sleep more refreshing and profound and increases the number of dreams.
• **Thyroid hormones:** people who lack these hormones are tired, forced to 'live' on their nerves and have difficulty sleeping at night.

● ● ● DID YOU KNOW?

> Prescribing hormonal medications and possibly giving hormone replacement therapy treatments is a matter for the doctor. Hormones are available only on prescription. Some hormones, such as melatonin, which has hit it big time in America, are not yet authorized to go on sale in Europe.

KEY FACTS

* Some hormones are involved in the sleep process.

* A deficiency of such hormones will disrupt your sleep.

* Tests can help ascertain and treat such deficiencies..

Chronic sleeping problems are often associated with neuroses, distress and discontent. Some treatments can be extremely effective but they are not always enough to control the fundamental problem. Your doctor can advise about medication or counselling.

49

give psychology a try

The adventurers of the forgotten past

Buried deep within our psyche, we all carry emotional scars that can be traced back to our childhood or adolescence. Most of the time we have forgotten the details of them. All that we have is the memory of the initial suffering. It is around these poles that we construct our intimate personality.

● ● ● DID YOU KNOW?

> Some therapies, particularly psycho-physical or emotional ones, are practised in groups. The dynamic that develops between the various participants forms an integral part of the healing process. You don't get better on your own but with the help of the other people, their emotions, their problems.

It sometimes happens that events that punctuate our lives find an echo in these early hurts, reawakening them – and us too, because our psychological and emotional problems can easily disturb our sleep. In that case there is just one solution: prepare to dive deep into yourself in search of the forgotten past.

The mind, the body, the emotions

To undertake this painful but sometimes necessary journey, you can gain support by communicating in a variety of ways.

• **Speech:** this is the tool used in traditional psychotherapy or psychoanalysis.

• **The body:** complementing the verbal exchanges with the therapist, some psychophysical therapies involve working on the body (such as dance, massage and breathing techniques).

• **The emotions:** there are processes that attempt to bring out the repressed emotions by any means, subsequently going on to work on material emerging so brutally from the subconscious.

• **Creativity:** other therapies try to go beyond mental barriers to help the person express themselves in a non-verbal way (through drawing, painting, writing or clay modelling, for example).

Each of these methods helps in its own way to uncover the intimate secrets and to relieve the patient of excessively heavy burdens. This helps improve sleep.

KEY FACTS

∗ Our history is often scarred by forgotten injuries which current events can reawaken and reactivate.

∗ In this case, it is necessary to go and explore the past to 'heal yourself'.

∗ Some therapies use speech, others the body, the emotions or creativity.

Whether taken on their own or as part of a course of therapy, flower essences can help you gently erase the scars of the past that cause you to suffer, especially those involving sleep-disturbing fears.

50

control your hidden fears

The mind and the body

Edward Bach (1886–1936) was a homeopath before he became interested in the 'soul' of the flowers (see pages 58–59). 'Even plants have therapeutic qualities that relieve human suffering,' he wrote. 'The ones I am looking for are real healing plants. Their task is not to relieve, but to heal, to restore health to the body and mind.' It's all a question of harmony.

● ● ● DID YOU KNOW?

> You can put a little of the essence (5 drops) in your bath water or massage a specific part of the body with about ten drops of undiluted essence.

> To improve sleep, massage either the solar plexus, an area that is often tense, or a more specific part of the body that is feeling tense (such as shoulders, back, nape of the neck).

Three essences to combat fears

• **You are in a panic** after a severe shock or intense stress. It is as though you are paralyzed, the only way you can react is with hysterical outbursts. Helianthemum (Rock Rose) will transform your fear into positive energy; you will once again be able to find the courage and control required to deal with emergency situations.

• **You are always extremely tense** as you are afraid of losing your self-control. You feel a great inner violence that remains hidden from other people. Prunus (Cherry Plum) will help you to express your feelings more easily and clearly and to find greater self-control.

• **You experience vague fears,** unspecified anxieties that plague your nights. Images, sometimes terrifying ones, appear. Your permanent feeling of insecurity makes you feel that you are always being watched, that you are 'host to a parasite'. Aspen will help you control your feelings without in any way making you materialistic. You will become more lucid and calm.

> Flower essences are available from some specialist pharmacies or in health food shops.

KEY FACTS

* Flower essences harmonize the relationship between the mind and the body to re-establish the conditions required for peaceful sleep.

* Some of these essences successfully combat the hidden fears that feed insomnia.

* You can also put the essences in your bath water or use them for a massage.

51
enjoy an ayurvedic massage

Derived from traditional Indian techniques, ayurvedic medicine tries to re-establish the balance between man and his environment. This therapy uses diet, meditation, plants and massage. Pleasure and effectiveness combined!

Disturbed harmony

Ayurvedic medicine is based on India's traditional ancient scriptures, the Veda. It endeavours to re-establish harmony between the body, the mental state and the mind in a relationship that is in balance with its environment. As in Chinese medicine, ayurveda believes that life materializes in the body in the form of an energy that flows through channels similar to the acupuncture meridians.

Any blockage of this energy, any psychological imbalance, any interruption to the harmony with the environment, can cause illness.

Preventative and curative massages

Massage is one of the most important therapies of ayurveda. Ayurvedic massage can be practised at home each day as a preventative measure. When performed by a specialist therapist, it can be curative and is particularly useful in treating entrenched insomnia.

Ayurvedic massage is carried out on the whole body starting with the feet, which give information on energy for the whole body. How the session then proceeds depends on the tensions that the masseur has detected beneath the arch of the foot. A specific vegetable oil is chosen to suit the person having the massage and their problems. These massages plunge the patient into a deep relaxation, unravelling the muscular knots and calming psychological tensions, whilst toning the body. You will sleep much better and wake feeling full of energy.

> *Shirodhara* is very effective in treating insomnia: a stream of tepid oil is poured onto the centre of the forehead, thus regulating the vital functions and calming the mind.

KEY FACTS

* Ayurvedic medicine is the traditional medicine of India.

* Massage is one of the techniques it uses.

* Whole-body massage calms physical and psychological tensions and improves sleep.

* Some local massages have a more specific function, some being specifically for sleep, for example.

52

unleash the power of aromatherapy

Essential oils are extremely concentrated plant extracts, much more powerful than the plants from which they are drawn. But they are also more dangerous and should therefore be handled with caution.

The wonderful world of aromas

Some plants, called aromatics, and some flowers contain substances that can be extracted by means of distillation. The composition of an essential oil differs from that of the original plant (see pages 52–53). Its extreme concentration of active constituents makes it into a very effective product but one that can be dangerous if taken orally. The prescribed dose must be adhered to right down to the precise number of drops.

Although essential oils should not generally be taken orally, some treatments, such as two drops of honey taken each evening in a teaspoon for two weeks, can be.

Anti-insomnia essences

- **For all types of insomnia:** marjoram, camomile, neroli, rosemary, lavender, mandarin, jasmine.
- **For anxiety-induced insomnia:** camomile, lemon balm, lime, vetiver, sandalwood, lavender, juniper.
- **If accompanied by depression:** basil, bergamot, jasmine, lavender, lemon balm, rosemary, orange, grapefruit, rose, citronella.
- **If insomnia is due to fatigue:** bergamot, cardamom, lemon, ginger, sage, verbena, thyme, fennel.

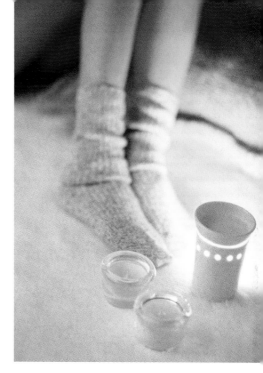

> In this case, the active constituents pass into the blood through the walls of the haemorrhoid veins, without having been altered by the digestive system.

 KEY FACTS

* Essential oils are extremely active plant concentrates.

* When taken orally, it is important to adhere to the prescribed dose because they can be toxic if the dose is exceeded.

* Some essences are soporific, others tranquilizing, antidepressant or tonic in effect.

53

Do a few minutes' yoga in the morning when you wake and at night before going to bed to relax you, banish depressing thoughts, calm the nervous system and stimulate hormonal secretions. You're guaranteed to sleep!

find out how yoga helps

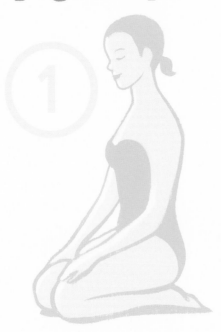

Reduce nervousness, increase hormone production

Yoga works on the body, respiration and concentration. It can also be used to promote self-awareness, to help you look at your inner self. This set of postures came into being around the 14th century BC in the Indus valley. Since then, yoga has travelled across the world. Research has shown that practising yoga regulates the neuro-vegetative system and stimulates the endocrine system, accelerating hormonal secretions, all of which leads to a rapid improvement in sleep.

Saluting the moon

Many postures can help put an end to insomnia and the moon salutation is one of them. You can do this posture morning and night.
① Kneel, then sit on your heels, with your hands on your thighs.

② Press your hands together in front of your chest, as though in prayer. Kneel up, put your right foot forward and place it on the ground in front of you.

③ Breathe in, then hold your arms out straight in front of you and breathe out. Breathe in again, then stretch your arms out to your side, level with your shoulders.

④ Breathe out, place your right hand on the ground by your right foot. Then breathe in, raise your head and look towards the sky. Breathe out and lower your head. Then return to position 2. Breathe out, place your left hand on the ground by your right foot, and proceed as for figure 4. Finally, return to the starting position.

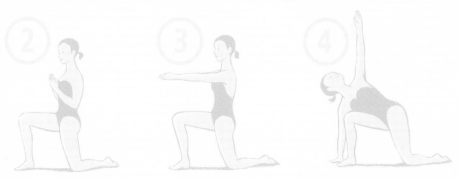

● ● ● DID YOU KNOW?

> It's best to do yoga at the same time and in the same place every day. Choose a quiet place where you will not be disturbed. It is best to do yoga on an empty stomach. Make sure you are lightly clad, so that your clothes do not get in the way, but you will not get too hot or too cold.

KEY FACTS

* Yoga is a work-out on the body, respiration and concentration, a chance to take a look at your inner self.

* It regulates the neuro-vegetative and endocrine systems, which improves sleep.

* Yoga needs to be practised at the same time and in the same place every day.

54

research trace elements

When insomnia has become entrenched and the body has become used to sleeping tablets, it is sometimes the case that natural treatments have hardly any effect in the short term. In this case, take food supplements to reinforce their effect.

Minute doses

When the body has become used to sleeping tablets for too long, insomnia can become resistant to natural treatments such as herbal and homeopathic remedies. In that case, using trace elements can increase the action of the herbal and homeopathic remedies. These mineral substances are present in the body in such minute amounts that they were long thought to be cellular metabolic waste. We now know that trace elements are essential for a whole host of biochemical reactions in the body. They act as a catalyst. Without them, reactions would occur inefficiently, if at all.

The brain and the nervous system

Some trace elements relate to the activity of the nervous system and the brain and, as a result, they have a role to play in the battle against insomnia. The most important trace elements in relation to insomnia are listed below:

• **You are stressed and irritable; you sleep only lightly and briefly:** take rubidium. This trace element stimulates the secretion of serotonin, the calm-inducing hormone, as well as acetylcholine and noradrenalin, two tranquilizing hormones.

> These treatments involve no risk of overdose or side effects.

• **You are depressed:** try copper-gold-silver. This mixture helps combat physical and particularly mental fatigue.
• **Your main problem is getting to sleep:** take manganese. It plays a fundamental role in the production of enzymes and hormones.
• **Lithium:** the Number 1 trace element for emotional and psychological problems. Lithium is used in conventional psychiatry to stabilize moods in manic depression. If used in significant amounts, regular blood tests are needed to avoid side-effects due to overdosage.

KEY FACTS

* Trace elements are minerals that are present in the body in minute amounts.

* They are essential catalysts for biochemical reactions.

* Some trace elements relate to psychological aspects and help relieve insomnia.

55

find out about medicinal plants

Phytotherapy (herbal medicine) is probably the oldest medicine in the world. And it still has a rosy future, especially in helping us to restore disturbed sleep. What's more, it causes fewer side effects than traditional medicine and there is no risk of addiction.

Infusion or decoction

Plants are living organisms which are often alive for only a short period of time. To get the most benefit from their healing properties, their active constituents must be preserved intact for as long as possible. A single plant contains many of these constituents which can act together to an even greater effect. Plants are traditionally used in the form of infusions or decoctions.

● ● ● DID YOU KNOW?

> Herbal remedies now come in various forms: blister packs, capsules, tablets. That way, they are easier to transport and more suitable for modern living.

> As a rule, capsules contain the whole plant, dried and powdered. Sometimes the plant is frozen to an extremely low temperature before being crushed.

To make an infusion, the dried plant is placed in boiling water and left to infuse for varying lengths of time. For a decoction, the plant is plunged into cold water and then boiled.

Plants for a good night's sleep

• **Black horehound:** although it is not really soporific, the black horehound is sufficiently calming to induce sound sleep, with no anxiety or nightmares.
To make an infusion: use 15 g per litre (1/2 oz per 1 3/4 pints) water. Leave to infuse for ten minutes. Drink the full amount during the course of the day.

• **Passionflower:** this is great against stress, very calming if you are overworked. If taken in large amounts, however, it can cause migraines. To make an infusion: use 1 tablespoon per cup of water. Leave to infuse for ten minutes. Never drink more than two cups a day.

> And finally, some methods of extraction using alcohol enable non-water-soluble active constituents to pass into the extract.

• **Hawthorn:** non-toxic, you need have no qualms about using hawthorn to treat distress. It quickly leads to good quality sleep. To make a decoction: use 10 g per 250 ml (1/3 oz per 8 fl oz) water. Boil for three minutes and then leave to infuse for ten minutes.

• **Bitter orange:** the flowers and leaves of the bitter orange tree have a calming effect and lead to sound sleep. To make an infusion: use 1 tablespoon per 1/4 litre (8 fl oz) water. Leave to infuse for ten minutes.

KEY FACTS

* Plants have been used to treat insomnia since time immemorial.

* They are effective, non-addictive and do not have side effects if taken correctly.

* Try black horehound, hawthorn, passionflower or bitter orange.

56

travel to China

Go on a tour of the Far East without leaving home: just follow the principles of Chinese medicine when choosing medicinal plants. Energy laws can also be applied to our own indigenous medicinal plants.

Five elements, five organs and five tastes

Plants are central to Chinese medicine, but Chinese doctors have a special way of choosing them. Like everything else that exists on this earth, plants have their own vital energy. Doctors decide the treatment for which they will be used on the basis of the property of this energy. In this way, each of the five main organs is symbolically linked with one of the five elements: Wood, Fire, Earth, Metal and Water. Depending on their individual taste, plants are also associated with these elements. Plants can be categorized as being yin (calming) or yang (stimulating).

Fire Yin plants

Insomnia is often due to an excess of energy in the heart meridian, and it is therefore often best to use Yin plants associated with Fire (the element linked with the heart) to restore calm, balance, harmony and sleep. Western plants such as hawthorn, passionflower and valerian can be included in this category. This comes as no surprise, as they are traditionally used in the West to treat insomnia. Less traditional, however, are marjoram, grape, lavender, sweet clover and mistletoe.

> All three forms are sometimes combined into a single energy extract, which is prepared in accordance with the principles of Chinese medicine.

KEY FACTS

* The Chinese use plants to treat medical complaints.

* The plants are chosen according to their energy properties.

* To treat insomnia, Chinese medicine usually recommends yin plants of the Fire element.

57 investigate anti-depressant plants

If your insomnia is due to depression, studies have shown that plant extract can be as effective as chemical anti-depressants, yet with fewer side effects. However, it does have significant interactions with conventional medications, including the contraceptive pill. Always take advice from a pharmacist.

The natural anti-depressant: St John's wort combats the symptoms of depression, including changes in sleep patterns. To promote regular sleep, take St John's wort extract, produced by macerating the plant in alcohol. This contains a sufficiently high proportion of hypericin, the active constituent responsible for the anti-depressant effect. Treatments range from 300 mg to 900 mg per day, depending on the severity of the depression.

Steer clear of mixtures

• If you are already taking anti-depressants, do not take St John's wort as well as your usual medication as hypericin is incompatible with certain molecules (in particular MAOIs).

• Do not suddenly stop taking an anti-depressant to replace it with St John's wort. Your symptoms could suddenly reappear with even greater severity.

• Consult a doctor to devise a plan for coming off an anti-depressant.

● ● ● D I D   Y O U   K N O W ?

> An analytical study of 1,757 patients found that 80% experienced some improvement in their depression over four weeks using St John's wort, whilst fewer than 20% experienced side effects (dry mouth, nausea, weight gain), compared with 50% when using chemical anti-depressants.

KEY FACTS

∗ Some changes in sleep pattern can be associated with depression.

∗ Extract of St John's wort has proved to be just as effective as chemical anti-depressants.

58 give biokinergy a whirl

A massage, micro-manipulation of the joints and energy investigation all rolled into one, biokinergy really does relieve chronic complaints, including insomnia.

An energetic massage: biokinergy is a massage technique developed in 1983 by the French physiotherapist, Michel Lidoreau. It is practised by specially trained physiotherapists. A special touch helps the biokinergist to make an energy 'assessment' and to locate areas where the joints, organs and especially the energy flows are blocked. The massage concentrates on certain points to remove all tensions (in the bones, tendons, muscles and organs), with the result that vital energy can flow freely.

Just two or three sessions are enough: each session lasts about an hour, the first one being the longest. Two or three sessions are usually all that's needed to treat insomnia. After that, you will just need a top-up session once a year to retain the benefits of the initial course of treatment.

KEY FACTS

∗ Biokinergy is a total massage technique.

∗ Areas of interest for biokinergy are osteo-articular statics, the organs and acupuncture points.

∗ It helps the body function harmoniously once again.

59

The Vittoz method helps combat stress and the problems it causes by re-educating our five senses – sight, touch, smell, taste and hearing. Insomnia is powerless against it.

explore the five senses

Act consciously

To re-learn how to sleep well, we have to silence our over-heated mind and rediscover our basic sensations. That is where our five senses come in. The founder of the method that bears his name, Dr Vittoz suggests that we feel rather than think: 'The exercise acts exactly where reason fails.'

He suggests daily exercises aimed at restoring our sensorial world to its rightful place. His main idea is to encourage us to do even the tiniest actions in our everyday lives consciously. This produces less stress, fewer parasitic thoughts, fewer mental and nervous tensions, a more harmonious inner life and better sleep.

Experience everyday actions to the full

Here are some examples of the most basic exercises to help make your five senses work:

• **Touch:** in the morning, brush your teeth feeling the brush in your hand, the bristles on your gums; note the noise you are making.

• **Smell:** before you put on your perfume, smell the open bottle; bring it up to your nostrils; then bring it back down towards the ground until the fragrance fades away.

• **Sight:** look at an object letting its image get right inside you, noticing even the tiniest details, the bumps, the irregularities

• **Taste:** when you eat something, let yourself be overwhelmed by the sensation it gives you and force yourself to make that sensation last as long as possible, even after you have swallowed it.

• **Hearing:** listen to a piece of music, following each instrument in turn.

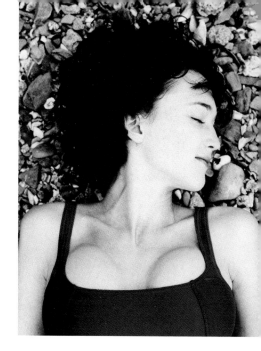

KEY FACTS

✳ The Vittoz method encourages you to learn to use your five senses consciously.

✳ Do the simple exercises every day to help silence parasitic thoughts.

✳ By improving the way in which we occupy space, we can offer a more effective resistance to the pressures that eat away at sleep.

60 encounter thalassotherapy

The sea spray of the beach, the treatments, the baths, the silence of the rest rooms, the flavours of healthy cooking – thalassotherapy is a package of treatments to promote deep relaxation and better sleep.

Have a tête-à-tête with yourself: the principle of thalassotherapy is simple – you spend a week tête-à-tête with yourself and you are entitled to five or six water-based treatments each day. You can alternate between jet showers, whirlpool baths, gymnastics in a heated swimming pool, underwater massage, mud baths, seaweed treatments and affusion showers to regain sound sleep.

Via the skin: the sea is very rich in all types of minerals and trace elements. Mud from the seabed laden with plankton and seaweed also has very high concentrations of micro-nutrients. Several studies have shown that these substances penetrate the body via the skin. Treatments also help relax the tensions that accumulate in the body.

● ● ● DID YOU KNOW?

> Many thalassotherapy centres also provide 'dry treatments' such as massage, relaxation, relaxation therapy and energy-flow medicine. So why not learn more, and with total peace of mind, about how these new measures can be used to combat stress and insomnia?

KEY FACTS

* Thalassotherapy involves making time for yourself.

* The micro-nutrients in seawater pass through the skin.

* Dry treatments (such as massage and relaxation therapy) help combat stress and restore sleep.

case study

I have started to live without medication

'I do a difficult job, which causes real nervous exhaustion. Two years ago, I had a trying year. I was always living on my nerves. I just could not sleep. I consulted a doctor who prescribed tranquilizers. Initially, I felt much better and I started to sleep again. But, before long, I had to increase the dose because the original one no longer had any effect. I began to be very distressed in advance at the idea of not having medication. It became an obsession: I always had to have two boxes of pills in store just in case…! It was my husband who put a stop to it. I wasn't aware that I was really addicted. My doctor drew up a plan to come off the tranquilizers, gradually replacing them with herbal remedies and trace elements.

I went through three difficult weeks, but now, I feel alive again. I sleep naturally; I wake up feeling full of energy in the morning; I don't spend hours huddled in bed trying to summon up the energy to start the day. Sheer bliss!'

useful addresses

» Acupuncture

British Acupuncture Council
63 Jeddo Road
London W12 9HQ
tel: 020 8735 0400
www.acupuncture.org.uk

British Medical Acupuncture Society
12 Marbury House
Higher Whitley, Warrington
Cheshire WA4 4QW.
tel: 01925 730727

Australian Acupuncture and Chinese Medicine Association
PO Box 5142
West End, Queensland 4101
Australia
www.acupuncture.org.au

» Homeopathy

British Homeopathic Association
Hahnemann House
29 Park Street West
Luton LU1 3BE
tel: 0870 444 3950

The Society of Homeopaths
4a Artizan Road
Northampton NN1 4HU
tel: 01604 621400

Australian Homeopathic Association
PO Box 430, Hastings
Victoria 3915, Australia
www.homeopathyoz.org

» Herbal medicine

British Herbal Medicine Association
Sun House, Church Street
Stroud, Gloucester GL5 1JL
tel: 01453 751389

National Institute of Medical Herbalists
56 Longbrook Street
Exeter, Devon EX4 6AH
tel: 01392 426022

» Massage

British Massage Therapy Council
www.bmtc.co.uk

Association of British Massage Therapists
42 Catharine Street
Cambridge CB1 3AW
tel: 01223 240 815

European Institute of Massage
42 Moreton Street
London SW1V 2PB
tel: 020 7931 9862

» Qi Gong

Qi Gong Association of America
PO Box 252
Lakeland, MN, USA
email: info@nqa.org

World Natural Medicine Foundation
College of Medical Qi Gong
9904 106 Street,
Edmonton AB T5K 1C4
Canada

» Relaxation therapy

British Autogenic Society
The Royal London
Homoeopathic Hospital
Greenwell Street
London W1W 5BP

British Complementary Medicine Association
PO Box 5122
Bournemouth BH8 0WG
tel: 0845 345 5977

» Yoga

The British Wheel of Yoga
25 Jermyn Street
Sleaford, Lincs NG34 7RU
tel: 01529 306 851
www.bwy.org.uk

acknowledgements

Cover: Hom/Stone; p. 8-9: M. Parmelee/Stone; p. 10, 15, 16, 21, 23, 24-25, 34-35, 40, 49, 52-53, 59, 88, 102-103, 104-105, 108-109: Neo Vision/Photonica; p. 12: P. Justin/Pix; p. 28-29: M. Dubois/Photonica; p. 31: Vital Pictures/Image Bank; p. 32: © Akiko Ida; p. 39: G. George/Pix; p. 43: R. Lockyer/Image Bank; p. 45: G. George/Pix; p. 51: © Akiko Ida; p. 57: S. Ozols/Image Bank; p. 60: G. George/Pix; p. 66: VCL/C. Tubbs/Pix; p. 68-69: M.Thomsen/Zefa; p. 71: G. & M.D. de Lossy/Image Bank; p. 77: R. Dunkley/Pix; p. 79: R. Lockyer/Image Bank; p. 83: M. Montezin and D. Eveque/Marie France; p. 86-87: V. Besnault/Pix; p. 93: D.R.; p. 94: Chassenet/BSIP; p. 97: J. Darell/Stone; p. 106-107: D.R.; p. 113: © Akiko Ida; p. 114-115: Photothèque/Hachette Livre; p. 117: M.Toi/Photonica; p. 121: B. Thomas/Stone.

Illustrations: p. 72-73, 74-75, 80-81, 98-99, 110-111: Marianne Maury Kaufmann; p. 4-5-6-18, 90-91: Laurent Rullier.

Editorial directors: Caroline Rolland and Delphine Kopff

Editorial assistant: Marine Barbier

Art editor: Guylaine Moi

Layout: G&C MOI

Final checking: Marie-Claire Seewald

Illustrations: Alexandra Bentz and Guylaine Moi

Production: Felicity O'Connor

Translation: JMS Books LLP